# The Inner Work *of* Birth

力

*Inner
Strength*

# The Inner Work of Birth

Nora Tallman, CNM

ISBN: 13: 978-15170005054
Printed in the U.S.A.

Published by Inner Work Press
2220 N. Country Club Drive
Canby, OR 97013

Photo credit: Page 124, Kelly Crull

# Dedication

This book is dedicated to my mother, Jean Tallman. She has given me one of the greatest gifts I have ever received—her unending love and support throughout my life. As I became a mother myself and strove to follow her example of maternal love, I experienced the sense of becoming a link in a chain. When I express to pregnant women that because of my mother, there has never been a moment in my life when I felt completely unloved, I sometimes see a look of pain cross their faces. My heart can feel that these are the women who didn't get a chance to experience that kind of relationship with their own mothers. I have learned to remind them that they can use their experiences to help guide them to make different choices, as they become mothers themselves. If they didn't receive unending maternal love, they can begin a chain of their own, to be passed on throughout the generations to come.

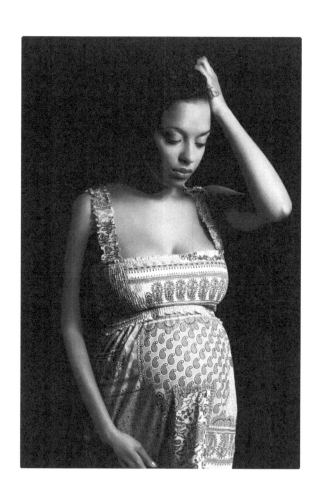

# Contents

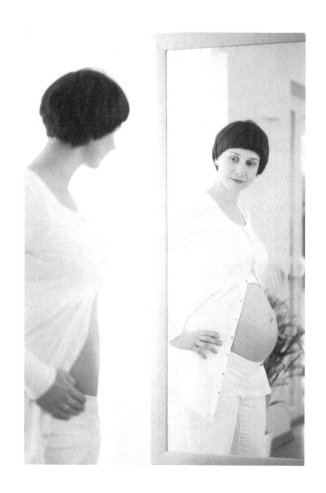

# Preface

I attended my first birth in 1978. Something resonated inside me and I began a long journey into the world of birthing. I trained with licensed midwives, naturopathic doctors, medical doctors, and certified nurse midwives. I spent years apprenticing and studying in academic and clinical settings. Most of the births I attended were in people's homes or freestanding birth centers until 2001 when I began exploring hospital birthing. By then I had also created a birth preparation class called "The Inner Work of Birth" that focused on emotional and mental preparation for birth. It was from the people that I served as a midwife, naturopathic doctor, and teacher that I learned the most about what birthing asks of women. Throughout this book I have included their words as italicized quotes that are insets within the text. It is a great gift to be allowed to share people's lives during such an intimate time.

Since the first twenty-three years of my midwifery career were spent doing out-of-hospital births, I have to admit that what I know best is natural birth. Mostly during those years I worked with people who were highly satisfied with their experiences and kept choosing natural birth for their subsequent babies. We transported about ten to twelve percent of our clients who encountered complications that required hospital interventions. As my interest grew in the internal experience of birth, I finally had to face the fact that I was working with a rather select group of women who were choosing out-of-hospital birth. The vast majority of babies in the United States are delivered in hospitals. How could I really understand what the birth experience was about without also working with women in a hospital setting? So, back to school I went and eventually ended up working in a hospital as a certified nurse midwife. Most of our clientele plan natural births and my interest continues in helping them to prepare for and have satisfying births. Whether a woman is birthing in or out of hospital, I still believe that her ability to access and utilize her own inner resources has a significant impact on her labor experience.

I began work on this book somewhere around the year 2000. Since then I have been gathering the material and exploring the concepts. I have found that many experienced birth attendants recognize and utilize emotional and mental components in the care that they provide. Some of what we do is instinctual and doesn't come from our logical brain. I have had to stretch myself in reaching enough clarity to formulate what has come to me through my feelings and through the emotional experiences of the people with whom I work. How do I describe the inspiration I have felt watching laboring women or the sadness in telling someone a week before their due date that I couldn't hear their baby's heartbeat through their abdomen? The more I pushed myself to formulate from both sides of my brain the more passionate I became about the inner world of birth.

# Introduction

This book is intended for people who are interested in natural birth. There are many books available that provide guidelines on how to get the birth you want. This book is different in that its focus is on preparing you to cope when you don't get what you want. For the vast majority of people on their journey through conception, pregnancy, laboring, birthing, breastfeeding, and parenting they will encounter at least one point, if not several, where reality does not match up with their expectations and desires. Sometimes we can have an influence on the course of our lives and sometimes we can't. What we really need to prepare for when bringing children into our lives are those hard times when we need to do what we don't think we're capable of. The transformation into parenthood often has its seeds in the effort to do what's needed instead of what we want. This is not being negative about birthing and childrearing. It's about honoring the effort as much as the joy of the whole experience.

One of my biggest challenges in creating this book is to write it in a manner that is free from any judgment about how women choose to birth. Natural birth isn't for everyone. I wish to state very clearly that women who choose to use pain medications during labor or elect to have cesarean deliveries have my complete support and respect. There is no wrong way to have a baby. A woman's freedom to choose what is right for her is a vitally important part of empowered birthing.

The challenge comes in describing the inspiration and gifts that can be part of natural birthing without implying that it is a more valid way to birth than one which utilizes medical interventions. This is particularly apparent when discussing the internal resistance that arises from intense pain, fatigue, or disappointment. This resistance is a normal part of natural birth. Yet, it is also a vulnerable time for laboring women. It is the point at which women often consider changing their original plans for an unmedicated birth. There is an art to knowing where to go in this situation. Is she asking for guidance and encouragement to push through her inner resistance and recenter herself back into coping or is she clearly communicating that she is done with that leg of the journey and is ready for an epidural? In that moment, my goal as a midwife is to try to decipher which pathway will bring her to the greatest satisfaction in the end. I've seen it go in many directions. If women choose to go on with natural birth I've seen them ecstatic that they didn't "give up" and have completed the journey as they intended. I've also seen women who were pressured into continuing on and end up feeling that they suffered through their natural birth. This is a fairly rare occurrence, but I am always sad to see it happen. If, instead, a woman chooses to have an epidural, there are still two outcomes that I have seen. Some women were delighted with their choice and felt that experiencing increased comfort and a chance to rest allowed them to enjoy the rest of their labor. On the other hand, I have also encountered women who come to me with their second pregnancy saying, "I was talked into an epidural on my first birth and I feel that I never got to experience all the parts of my labor. This time I want to stick with my plan for a natural birth." Ultimately, it is always a woman's choice, but many times it is not an easy decision in the moment.

This book could be valuable to people who see their lives as a journey of self-exploration and growth. Within the context of the maternity experience, it explores finding your courage when you're worried or anxious. It looks at the incredible challenge of releasing control in a situation that means so much to you. It discusses ways to call up your power when you're feeling helpless. It honors the peace and strength that can be found in acceptance. In the end, my goal is that your satisfaction is not dependent on getting the birth you want. My hope is that I can help you want the birth you get.

力

# Acknowledgements

I wish to express my gratitude to the many fellow midwives and other birth attendants with whom I have shared the world of birthing. We've connected through laughter and tears. We understand each other in a way that no one else can. We know that when a phone rings at 3:00 in the morning, it gets answered because we're always there when we're really needed. I must mention Catherine and Penni because you both have been with me through so many of the experiences that have shaped this book.

My sincere thanks goes to those faithful souls who read through the first drafts of these pages and gave me feedback. These especially include Gina and Kathy. I could not have chosen a better editor than Deirdre, who is the comma queen, and who polished my words into a quite presentable final text. The finishing touch came with my book designer, Gillian, whose artistry with space, color and fonts helped bring my work to its final stages.

The support I received from my family kept me going through a fifteen-year book labor. Mom and Aric, my heart will always come home to you. And my list of gratitudes would not be complete without including my horse, Tessa, and our trainer, Karen. With your help I am balanced and restored.

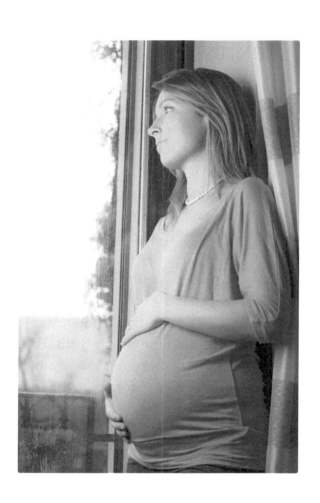

力

# Preparing for Empowered Birthing

*Everything in life prepares
a woman for labor.*

One of the first steps in getting ready for birthing is to recognize that you're already well on your way. You've spent years maturing into the woman that you are today. Everything in life prepares a woman for labor. It is a matter of validating your previous experiences and understanding how they relate to what you will need when you give birth. When you tried out to be a cheerleader, you exerted courage to take a risk. When you made it through four long years of college, you developed perseverance and determination. When you took off traveling, you practiced self-reliance. When you faced your boyfriend falling in love with someone else and announcing your relationship was over, you made it through surviving when you didn't get what you wanted. And if you have never experienced any of these examples, you have encountered many other challenges that are equally valuable. Even if you are facing labor for the first time, you still come to it with your own inner strengths and capabilities. These are the best resources that you could have.

✦

ABOUT TEN YEARS AGO, *my partner and I broke up after five years of being in a relationship. Unfortunately, we were on an island in Thailand at the time where I had no friends or support. Fortunately, I relied on myself in a way I had never done before. I grieved the relationship, but somehow managed to make new connections with people and then continued to travel around the world for five more months on my own. It was a birth of sorts for me.*

✦

IN THE "INNER WORK OF BIRTH" *group we were talking about where we imagined we could give up in labor. I realized that I had been identifying myself as physically weak. I imagined not having stamina, strength, being unable to deal with pain, and having to give up. I then had a chuckle inside and thought, "How could that be?" I have not always identified as being so physically weak. I then remembered my growing-up years, living in a town that was 99% Italian Catholic and having a Jewish background. I remembered all of the anti-Semitism I had to deal with and, particularly, when I beat up the gang leader. A group of girls waited for me after school one day, ready to get me. I walked through them as they pushed me, and then the leader came and began a more serious confrontation. I punched her in the face, she fell to the ground, and I ran onto the school bus. Remembering that experience put me in contact with the street fighter in me; the one who was strong and could meet difficult experiences.*

Another important piece of birth preparation is recognizing the role that participation plays in bringing you to a place of high self-satisfaction. When you are planning for a natural birth, it is helpful to see value in the effort that it will require of you. Knowing that you have given your best effort is linked to your satisfaction. Sometimes obstacles occur that may change where you thought you were going and sometimes the journey is not what you thought it would be. Unexpected events do not have to change your ownership of your experience when you continue to participate to the best of your ability.

✦

A FEW YEARS BEFORE I GAVE BIRTH, *I walked a marathon. By mile twenty I was excited because I only had six more miles to go. Those last six miles were just taking one foot and putting it in front of the other. To me, stopping wasn't an option. Labor was the same experience, one breath at a time. Remembering that every contraction brought me closer to crossing the finish line helped me to get through it all.*

✦

IN SOME WAYS BIRTH REMINDED ME *of some of my previous extreme physical challenges: like pounding in two-hundred tomato stakes in a California field in ninety-five degree weather, or biking for days on end, or hiking up a mountain with a huge pack on. Those things are difficult physically, but what made the birthing experience a unique challenge for me was that I had no idea what was happening or how long it would go on, or how strong it would get. But I do think that doing things that are challenging physically and emotionally helped prepare me somewhat for birth.*

## Influencing the Perception of Pain

Understanding where and how you have choices is an important part of full birthing participation. Since coping with pain is such a significant challenge in a natural birth let's look at where you have choices about it. It's tempting to look for ways that will make the pain less intense. Using water, massage, or position changes may decrease the discomfort when the contractions are still relatively mild in early labor. Then, when active labor starts (usually when the cervix is dilated about five to six centimeters) the contractions increase in intensity. It is important to recognize that the contractions in early labor are not strong enough to complete cervical dilation in active labor. As the hours pass, it is like going up the steps of a staircase with each step bringing stronger contractions. This is normal labor. Telling your body to not bring on these bigger contractions is sending it a message to stall out in labor. You might want to say instead: "Bring it on—let's do this efficiently!"

With the stronger contractions of active labor the challenges of coping also increase. External measures to decrease the intensity of the pain are often not enough if you are struggling internally to stay afloat. This is when something more is needed. Describing the physiology of pain perception helps to clarify how you can shift your internal state back into coping.

✦

WE NEED A DIFFERENT WORD THAN PAIN *to describe the sensation of contractions. Pain is like scraping your knee—that sharp, stinging feeling. Contractions are more than pain.*

There are two components in your body that are activated when you experience pain. During labor, nerve endings get pressed on and send messages up the spinal cord to the brain. Then, the emotional center in the brain interprets these messages and gives them meaning. This is where you have a choice about how you perceive the pain. You can object to the sensations, seeing them as wrong. This response decreases your ability to cope and leaves you resisting what is happening. The alternative is to choose to agree with the sensations, accepting them. When you do this you are working with the labor process and coping with the pain. Coping with pain is not about changing the sensation. It is about changing your attitude about the pain and thus allowing you to respond effectively. The place where you have influence over pain is how you interpret and relate to it.

*Coping with pain is not about changing the sensation. It is about changing your attitude about the pain and thus allowing you to respond effectively.*

✦

THE PRESSURE, THEN THE BURNING, THE HEAD EMERGING, *and then the shoulders, and then the slippery and fast whoosh of my new baby from my body. So much effort and pain of labor and then its whole body just slides out with such little effort and pain. It reminds me that making a baby really happens beyond our control, and it happens so perfectly, so beautifully, with relatively little effort for such an incredible creation.*

# Utilizing All of Who You Are
# in the Birthing Process

Many people agree that we are made up of at least three different "centers": *body*, *heart*, and *mind*. Many would also add a fourth as the *spiritual center* that will be discussed more in the next chapter. All of these parts have their roles in supporting the birthing process.

In preparing for birth many women rely on the belief that their body will know what to do when labor starts. It is rather magical to realize that your uterus knows how to contract, open up, and push your baby out of your vagina. In the birthing process the physical body leads the way. It is helpful to trust that it knows how to birth a baby even if your mind doesn't get the picture.

Your body will usually know how to do labor, but it isn't so great at knowing how to cope with labor—that's the job of the heart and the mind. Both centers need to support the body as it proceeds in one of the greatest tasks you will ever take on in your life. People talk about "cutting off your head" in labor in order to allow your body to do its work. The problem with this approach is that your heart and mind are abandoning your body when it needs you the most. If you attempt to disassociate from the painful sensations of labor you remove the support that your body so desperately needs. If, instead, you accept and appreciate the sensations, all of your centers are activated and you birth with the whole of your being. Then, the challenge of labor becomes doable. With your mind, you focus the healing power of attention, perceiving each of the contractions without judgment. With your heart, you wish your body well and send gratitude for the work that it is so willingly taking on.

*Your body will usually know how to do labor, but it isn't so great at knowing how to cope with labor—that's the job of the heart and the mind.*

✦

*My body, my soul—I sometimes feel that they are not connected with my mind. In labor, they connected. My mind kind of stopped thinking in "reality." It focused in on my body. Communicating with people was really hard; my mind was turned inward and didn't want to be brought out. I felt my whole self.*

All of your centers have the capability of either supporting or hindering the birth process. The following are examples of how this might manifest. Your body can accept the sensation of contractions, leading to relaxation; or, it can resist them, causing tension. Your heart can be grounded, creating a sense of calmness verses reacting dramatically, which can lead to a feeling of distress. Your mind can maintain a clear picture of your overall aim in birthing your baby, which connects you with your ability to adapt if unexpected events arise. This is in contrast to your mind being distracted by unintentional associative thoughts that are fertile ground for becoming overwhelmed in worry. You have a much higher chance of creating the birth experience that you desire if you are doing all that you can to make intentional choices from each of your centers.

## Intentional Choice to Birth Naturally

Women have been birthing babies for many thousands of years. While much has changed in the external events surrounding birth, fundamentally we have the same bodies and experience the same physical process as women who lived, for instance, five thousand years ago. They had the same nerve endings that we have, and we share the same job of getting our babies born. However, there are some significant differences in how we process the experience internally now. Ancient women were probably much more accustomed to experiencing extreme effort, discomfort, and tedious work than most of us are today. Let's face it—we live easier lives! The kind of work that it takes to birth a baby without pain medications is relatively unique compared with our daily lives. Our ancient sisters were also probably much more familiar with chronic pain. They could have suffered with a tooth abscess for years while we just have to make it through until we can get a dentist appointment.

Given that so many more women and babies died during birth or soon after, ancient women were much more concerned about survival than we are now. While there are certainly still parts of the world where this continues to be a significant issue, most women with access to modern medicine face a very remote possibility of fatal harm to themselves or their babies. Modern technology has good solutions for the three main causes of maternal complications: hemorrhage, blood pressure problems, and infection. These treatments for pregnant women, along with resuscitation and advances in managing preterm and sick babies, have also dramatically improved the outcome for babies. There is no question that these advances save many lives. Being freed up of some of the concerns for survival, the modern woman has more time to focus on the quality of her birth experience and a greater sense of being able to make choices.

*Being freed up of some of the concerns for survival, the modern woman has more time to focus on the quality of her birth experience and a greater sense of being able to make choices.*

One of the choices that you face today is whether to birth naturally or to use medical interventions, particularly pain medications. While complications may require interventions, how you deal with the pain of labor is still mostly your decision. Ancient women did not have to make this choice. In the midst of full labor, they never had to wonder, "Should I get an epidural now or do I choose to keep going on my own?" Their reason for laboring naturally was simply to get their babies born. That was their only pathway. The modern woman now has to make an intentional choice to birth naturally. This is only something that has come up for most laboring women in the last century. This existence of a new choice has had a profound impact on a women's internal experience of birthing. Intentional choice requires developing a motivation that comes from within you. It also means that there is flexibility built into it so that you maintain your freedom to change your course if that is what is best for you.

## Building an Effective Motivation for Birthing

One of the most effective ways to prepare yourself for labor is to clearly formulate what motivates your intentions for a natural birth. What motivates you to make this choice? Throughout my years in midwifery, I have asked thousands of women this question. The most common answer that I have heard is that they are planning a natural birth because they want to avoid medical interventions. When asked why they want to avoid medical interventions they usually explain that they don't like them, don't trust them, or they are afraid of them. They often see interventions as taking over control of the birth process and adding the potential for complications that can cascade into an impersonal, dehumanized experience. Information from the media and friends often promotes natural birth based on an aversion to the medicalized approach of Pitocin, epidurals, and cesarean deliveries.

◆

> MY GREATEST FEAR WAS INTERVENTION: *to interrupt or alter the natural, forceful, subtle, incomprehensible process of labor and delivery seemed to me like trying to change the weather or the tides. At best, daring; at worst, deeply dangerous.*

Researchers such as Elliot and Gable (2006, 2010) have studied the psychological models of approach verses avoidance motivation. They have consistently shown that people are more able to achieve their goals when they focus on where they want to go instead of what they want to avoid. My years of experience as a midwife have verified that the avoidance motivation described in the previous paragraph does, indeed, come with significant problems and is often ineffective. If you are choosing natural birth primarily because you want to avoid interventions you may end up making the interventions the enemy who is lurking around the corner. This can magnify your fear and increase your concerns about danger and things going wrong. If the birth process doesn't progress normally or safety issues arise, interventions may become necessary. Then you end up facing what you wanted to avoid and having to ask it for help. You run the risk of interpreting this as a failure or seeing yourself as a victim. A third problem

*People are more able to achieve their goals when they focus on where they want to go instead of what they want to avoid.*

with depending on an avoidance motivation is that it often isn't effective when you encounter the really big challenges in labor. Trying to find your inner strength when you're running away from something creates an internal contradiction. It may be more helpful to cultivate internal states that bring you energy rather than drain you.

A more effective approach is to build a positive motivation for choosing to birth naturally. Ask yourself: "What experience am I seeking when I choose to birth this way?" This approach has much more of a sense of moving towards something. One suggestion is to formulate what you wish for as an internal experience and leave the external events some flexibility in how they might play out. Remember that the place where you have the most influence is inside yourself. Your motivation needs to be in your own words and come from what you value as an individual. Areas that you might want to think about are viewing the birth experience as a potential opportunity for self-growth or discovering parts of yourself that you don't know much about. Finding out about your own strengths and capabilities is extremely valuable as you transform into a parent. Birthing with your partner may provide explorations into your relationship and broaden what you share together. These are the kinds of motivations that you can hang onto if you feel overwhelmed with pain or fatigue or you are facing an unexpected event and it feels like all your plans are collapsing. Some part in you can keep moving forward no matter what is happening on the outside.

I'VE NEVER DONE ANYTHING IN MY LIFE *that was really important all by myself. I'm about to become a mother and I don't know that I have the strength or capability to be a good mother. I want to experience those qualities in my labor so that I will know that I can count on myself when my baby needs me.*

✦

I WANT TO FEEL CONNECTED *to my baby, body, and the whole birth experience. I want to give myself the opportunity to be extraordinary. I also dislike the idea of not having some element of control; although this is less of an issue now because I can think of ways to reframe what "control" means. Finally, I feel like I can be more involved if we try for a natural/low-intervention childbirth.*

✦

BEFORE TAKING THE "INNER WORK OF BIRTH" *class I hadn't really thought of why I wanted to have a natural birth. After going through the class I've learned more about myself and why the way I birth matters to me. I feel like a natural birth is a way I can learn more about myself and grow. I want to be proud of myself and feel excited about my accomplishment. I think that birth is going to be a grounding experience in the sense of feeling close to the basic way of doing things. I also want to feel connected to other women who have done this and to nature. It seems like an experience that pulls energy from the trees and stars. I want to work **hard** at this!*

Once you are clear on what it is that you wish for in your birth experience, how can you prepare to make it happen? When you place your focus on your inner motivation you expand your capability to cope with what is happening on the outside. The rest of this book explores the process of the inner work of birth. Chapters four through seven are in depth discussions of four important components of a fulfilling birthing experience. These can be summarized as:

1. **Find the truth.** This requires your courage to acknowledge your fears and illusions in order to see the reality both about yourself and the situation that you are in.

2. **Make the choice.** This necessitates your willingness to experience what is happening.

3. **Create the freedom.** This needs your acceptance of the situation even if it means you may not be getting what you want.

4. **Trust yourself and your own capabilities.** This calls for your effort to do what needs to be done.

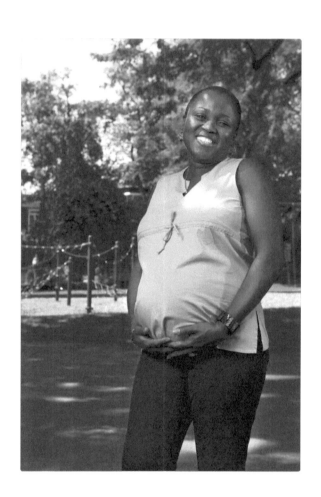

力

# Transformation and Sense of Self

*We become the choices that we make.*

The coming of a baby into your care, particularly a first baby, brings with it not only major changes in your lifestyle, but also a deep influence on your sense of who you are. One day you are pregnant and the next day you are enmeshed in breastfeeding, diapers, soothing your baby's cries, and gazing in wonder at his or her sleeping face. As the days pass, your role as a mother or father emerges from within. It is sometimes challenging for people to really believe how much something outside themselves could change their lives. When the hurricane of parenthood hits it can take a lot of trust on your part that you will end up whole when the air finally clears. What was once new and unfamiliar, with time, becomes a comfortable part of how you see yourself in the world. This time of transformation from pregnancy into parenthood is rich with potential for becoming more of who you wish to be.

✦

THE BEST THING ABOUT BECOMING A PARENT *is discovering that your capacity to love another person is so much deeper than you ever imagined it could be.*

✦

*I'VE BEEN AMAZED AT HOW QUICKLY I CHANGED from being concerned with time and how long activities were taking, to not worrying about time being wasted. I used to hate getting out of bed late—I loved being up early and getting my day started. Now I want to spend time in bed with my baby. I also love it when my baby takes his time to nurse; the longer the better! I'll happily gaze into his eyes or stroke his back and hair. I find myself just watching him when I should be doing housework, and I feel happy. I don't feel stressed or annoyed that I'm "wasting time."*

Transformation is a process that moves from a stable state (how things are) through a formless space of chaos and out into a new form (how things will be). Even if your life wasn't perfect before pregnancy, at least you generally knew what to expect most days. Once you are pregnant, it's not just your body that changes. Parts deep inside you are already shifting in preparation for what will come. It becomes necessary to adapt what were once familiar parts of your lifestyle to accommodate the needs of your pregnancy. You begin serving your baby many months before he or she is born. The transformation is most dramatic during labor and birth. It is helpful to recognize that birth's intensity is part of the chaos that is necessary to take apart the old in the process of creating the new. It's not just a baby that is being born. The role formation of mother and father has a very significant impact on who you are. Even if it's not a new role for you, you have never parented this child before, and he or she may have a profound impact on your family structure.

*Once you are pregnant, it's not just your body that changes.*

✦

*FOR ME, PARENTING PRESENTS the continual challenge of being in the moment, expecting and accepting the unexpected. Being present with my son means being less attached to outcomes. It challenges me to be patient and flexible with myself and those around me. I see now that I have tended to value outcomes over process in some areas of my life. My son has taught me that knocking down is as important as building up.*

BIRTH CHANGED ME *in that it was intense physically, but also emotionally. I have cried more times from tenderness and joy in the past nine months than I have in years. I have become more connected to my emotions, needs, and desires since giving birth. Parenting (so far) has been humbling. It has changed the way I look at life. No longer just "mine" but now my daughter's—she plays a huge part in my daily life. This is a huge, huge adjustment. I'm learning to act with compassion and patience more often... to slow down the pace of life.*

There are many examples of the changes that women face as they move through pregnancy and into motherhood. Some women report that fatigue or a shift in focus or interest decreases their effectiveness in their work or school life. Their growing pregnant bodies may diminish their ability to move quickly or sustain athletic activity. Particularly for women who have spent a significant part of their adult life developing a career and earning their own money, it can be a big adjustment to stay at home and be supported financially, even if it's only for a few months. Probably the most common change that women describe with new motherhood is a decrease in personal freedom. Serving the needs of a newborn is a full time job that doesn't stop when the sun goes down. Especially in the first three months, there isn't much of a break. Two hundred years ago women didn't have much opportunity to experience an independent adult life without the responsibility of caring for children. They tended to move from their parents' home into the homes they shared with their husbands. Motherhood often followed quickly. Today's women are more likely to have spent several years to decades living independently as adults before deciding to bring children into their lives. Nothing will alter their lifestyle more than adding a baby to the house. For example, it will affect their sleep, how they spend their time and money, how they will relate to their breasts, the ease with which they will make a trip to the grocery store, and what they will do for entertainment.

AFTER MY DAUGHTER WAS BORN, *I laid with her in my arms. I had needed a cesarean delivery since my placenta had implanted between my baby's head and the opening to the uterus. Despite all that was wrong, the baby in my arms was so right. My mom and sister kept trying to get me to put the baby in the nursery so I could sleep. The thought panicked me. I couldn't let her go away from me, but held her as I slept. Once, I woke to my sister trying to lift her away from my body. I was enraged that she would take her from me. I felt like a mother wolf, some kind of animal that would protect my baby no matter what the consequence to myself. I figured I would catch up on my sleep once I was home. I was wrong. It was the beginning of a couple years of sleep depravation.*

Babies relate to their mothers' bodies not only as a source of food, but their touch is a source of comfort. Intimacy before children usually has sexual overtones. With motherhood you learn how your body can connect with another human being in a totally new way. This new sense of the link between your body and your heart may have some influence on your lover relationship with your partner. Most couples report that the frequency of sexual contact decreases in the months after their baby is born. This is largely due to fatigue and a simple lack of time. Yet, there is also a readjustment that needs to happen as couples explore how the transformation into parenthood has affected them both as lovers.

I KNEW THAT THIS WOULD BE THE BIGGEST CHALLENGE I *have faced thus far in my life, and now being on the other side of the experience, it is the thing I am most proud of. When I look in the mirror now, I see my body very differently. I have a new appreciation for every curve and soft spot, as I know these are parts of the body that delivered my baby. But, it wasn't just my body that did all of the hard work; it was so much my state of mind and my ability to trust myself as well as my husband and my midwife.*

While all of these external life changes may feel a bit chaotic, they also offer opportunities for internal transformation. When our lives begin shifting and rapidly changing it is useful to ask ourselves: "What is it I really want in my life and who do I want to be?" While we can't control many of the changes that pregnancy, birthing, and parenthood bring; we always have a choice in how we respond internally to the external events around us. Our part in creating who we are is that we become the choices that we make.

✦

I SUPPOSE IT'S STILL EARLY, *but I can definitely sense a further detachment from my intellect, which has dominated decision-making and emotion throughout my life. Since marrying my husband, the intuitive side has slowly emerged; and now, with the birth of our son, it is in the driver's seat. There is a sense of simultaneous fear and exultation at ceding to this intuition.*

## The Boundaries of Your Sense of Self

Your sense of self is the image with which you define yourself in life. It is what you use to differentiate who you are verses who someone else is. Psychologically it is made up of your individual beliefs, attitudes, expectations, values, buffers, and habits. Your sense of self often guides you on an unconscious level so that you don't stop to think what an appropriate response might be in a conversation or what action to take when you feel something isn't right. Without a sense of self you wouldn't be able to function on a daily basis. Everything would be brand new and you would have no internal reference structure to use when making the multitude of choices that living requires of you. A simple example would be brushing your teeth every morning. You might believe that this activity promotes dental health and prevents foul-smelling breath. You feel that this is a valuable thing to do, and, besides, you've been brushing your teeth every morning for as long as you can remember. You have just utilized a belief, a value, and a habit to decide on what action to take while standing there in front of the sink.

✦

> I DIDN'T EXPECT MY BIRTHING EXPERIENCE *to be so much like my personality and style of adapting to change; but it was. Slow to start labor, coming on really strong once it got started, wanting to stop when it got too overwhelming. I didn't believe that I could do it or that it was over!*

It is useful to have a clear understanding of what these parts of your sense of self are. Additionally, ask yourself the following questions to help identify your own internal references for coping with labor. (The first one—what you value—is so critical to the choices you make in childbirth that it is discussed in more depth in the next chapter):

1. **A value** is what you hold as important or useful. *How important is it to you to fully participate in your baby's birth?*

2. **A belief** is something that the mind has accepted as true. It is what you largely use to differentiate what is real from what is false. *What do you believe you are capable of when it comes to meeting the challenges of labor?*

3. **An attitude** is more emotionally-based and is a feeling or an opinion about something. *How do you feel about experiencing intense, painful sensations?*

4. **An expectation** is a sure belief or intense hope that something will happen in a particular way. *What should your birth look like?*

5. **A buffer** is used to soften an impact or protect yourself from an undesired effect. *How honest are you with yourself in acknowledging what the birth may ask of you?*

6. **A habit** is a pattern of something you repeatedly do that is often unconscious. *What role do you often take when you are in a stressful situation?*

As you were growing up you began developing the capability to think and act independently. You started to make choices for yourself in response to what life sent your way. From true friendships you may have developed a trusting nature while an experience of rejection may have caused you to choose caution as an effective survival tool. By the time you reached adulthood much of your sense of self had firmed up into a form that you identify as being who you are. Often without realizing it, you have spent your life forming the parts of your sense of self. Mostly you function on an unconscious level when you utilize these parts to make the multitude of choices that your daily life requires.

Fortunately, not all of the decisions that you make are unconscious. You also have the capacity to make intentional choices. In fact, some of these choices may even challenge the boundaries of your sense of self and change it into something else. This is the basis of personal growth.

✦

> THE BEST AND MOST USEFUL THING ABOUT PREGNANCY AND PARENTING *is that it slowed me down. I've always been an on-the-go kind of person and my nausea in pregnancy would not let me do that. Then, once we had our child, it was like all of the clutter and crap in my life just vanished. From the second I laid eyes on my son, my priorities got in line. Now I have this even richer, more beautiful life of connection with my family and the world around me. The pace of being present to another human being is very slow. For the first year of my baby's life, I described myself as having a very small outer life (no new clothes, travels, vacations, social nightlife), but a huge inner life (in awe of life, deep belly laughs, and being a part of another human's development).*

Your values, beliefs, attitudes, expectations, et cetera, form the boundaries that contain your sense of self. A boundary is formed when you decide that you believe this and you don't believe that; this is valuable and that isn't. You need some kind of internal form in order to be able to function mentally and emotionally. It becomes interesting when you start questioning if certain boundaries are useful for security or have they become the walls of your self-created prison? When life asks more of you than you feel capable of, can you choose inner freedom, break through a boundary and become who you need to be? This kind of inner effort is how you participate in the creation of yourself—allowing you to grow more into the human being that you wish to be.

An example of this might be a woman who doesn't want to push hard enough to get her baby born because she can't bear the thought that she might push stool out of her anus in front of everyone attending her birth. Her belief that she is not a woman who can defecate in front of other people is getting in the way of doing what she needs to do. She is struggling with a self image, a sense of appropriate behavior regarding what is private and what is acceptable to do in the company of others, perhaps a judgment that poop is disgusting and embarrassing. We can reassure her that, as birth attendants, we clean up laboring women's poop all the time and that it is no big deal to us. That doesn't matter; it's still a big deal to her. What she is facing is an internal boundary that only she can choose to break through. In this situation, she can choose the freedom to be someone that she previously didn't believe she could be.

✦

> EVEN THOUGH I WAS READY FOR PUSHING, I KIND OF FROZE UP. *I was suddenly very scared of pooping or peeing in front of everyone, and I was still having a hard time understanding that the feelings I was having were really going to push out that baby. I was feeling the urge to push, but it wasn't enough to overcome my fears. After being convinced some more by everyone, I was able to start pushing, but I'm not sure that I was making much progress.*

In preparing for your baby's birth, it's useful to spend time searching for more recognition of your own inner boundaries, especially those that you might encounter during labor. What beliefs do you hold about what is acceptable and what isn't? What do you expect will happen, and could you cope if something else occurred instead? How do you habitually respond when you are really tired and you still have to keep working? What do you tell yourself to get out of things you don't want to do?

Sometimes the boundaries that might stop you in labor come from inside yourself and sometimes they are a result of an external event over which you have no control. For example, how you respond to the pain of labor is an internal choice while how easily the baby descends into your vagina is a function of the size and position of your baby, the strength of the contractions, and the shape of your pelvis. Understanding where you have choices and where you don't allows you to focus your efforts on the boundaries where you have a chance of having an influence.

When you encounter an internal boundary, emotionally it feels like you've hit up against a wall. It may feel solid; immovable—it's just how things are. The first step in working with a boundary is to step back and identify its nature and to formulate the message that it is sending you. For instance, during labor you may hold the belief that you work best alone and don't need help from others. The second step is to question its reality. If you have been inwardly withdrawn and find yourself feeling stuck in labor, is this a circumstance where working

*Understanding where you have choices and where you don't allows you to focus your efforts on the boundaries where you have a chance of having an influence.*

alone is what serves you best? Is it true that you are incapable of asking for help or is the truth that you don't usually make a habit of turning to others for assistance? The last step is to make a choice about continuing to work with the boundary the way it is or to change it. Many of your internal boundaries are only illusions that mostly exist below your level of consciousness. They're not as absolute as you take them to be. In the example above, you could choose to turn to your birth attendant and say, "I need help; I don't feel like I'm going anywhere in this labor and I don't know what to do." This may be something that you're not accustomed to vocalizing, but you can find the courage to ask if the need is great enough. Sometimes your inner boundaries are not an obstacle for you— instead, they are exactly what you need to pull you through. It may be that when it comes to pushing in labor, you may choose to maintain your strong sense of self reliance and find it a great aid in effectively moving your baby down your vagina and into your waiting arms.

✦

*I HAD ALTERNATIVELY CLIMBED STAIRS and used a breast pump in order to keep labor going for hours—the whole time praying for the contractions to come harder. When I got to the edge of the cliff and the labor was really happening—when I really had to relinquish control—I met resistance. I was in so much pain, and I really didn't think I could do it. My mind didn't think I could. It all seemed far too much to do. After a few contractions of trying to weasel out of it—saying I couldn't do it—that it was too much, my midwife just looked me straight in the eyes and said, "This is where you have to choose. You can't think about it. You have to take a spiritual leap and trust your body." Just like that I was back in my body, choosing with my body, not my mind; letting go. I had to let go with my mind and just be in my body fully. It didn't stop hurting, but I was no longer resisting. I was fully engaged in the utterly physical work of birth—which is the most spiritually-alive thing I'll ever do. Within an hour my son was born.*

The essence of birth requires breaking through boundaries. On a physical level this manifests mostly in your body. Your sense of who you are in the material world is usually defined as the edge where your skin contacts air. During pregnancy, that boundary changes shape dramatically and you take up more space. Your body also forms the edge of your baby's home as it grows inside. The opening to the uterus stays tightly closed to keep your baby in place until labor begins. Then, in a matter of hours, the passageway has to get bigger as the cervix opens to allow the baby to move from its internal environment, through the boundary of your body and out into the world to begin an independent life.

*The essence of birth requires breaking through boundaries.*

Mentally and emotionally there are also many boundaries that meet resistance and are then transformed. Your level of physical contact with anyone besides your partner often dramatically changes during and after pregnancy. During pregnancy your body is examined more frequently than usual and afterwards you will spend countless hours in contact with your baby as you nurse and carry him or her. It doesn't stop when a baby starts walking on his or her own. Most mothers have many years of children crawling all over them as they relate to their bodies as places of comfort and security. Your boundary of your sense of self will be enlarged to incorporate your role as a mother. Many beliefs concerning what you thought you were capable of will transform as you serve the needs of gestating, birthing, and raising a child. One of the most wonderful boundaries that grows is your capacity to love your baby beyond anything you have experienced before.

◆

> PREGNANCY WAS A VERY HEALING EXPERIENCE *for me in that it changed my relationship with my body in a positive way. Having struggled with an eating disorder for many years and never feeling completely comfortable in my own skin, I was surprisingly able to relax into myself while pregnant and appreciate the beauty, power, and capability of my body as it grew life.*

Your internal boundaries are often unknown. It would be difficult to describe more than a small part of who you believe yourself to be. You learn more about your boundaries when you're pushed up against them. Birthing may offer you chances to bring parts of yourself that you don't know well into a spotlight. Labor and birth may push you to the edge of yourself, and then often requires you to go farther.

## The Spiritual Aspect of Birthing

Birth can be seen as a spiritual journey when you view it as an opportunity to discover more about yourself and to grow into your potential. Its challenges call on your strengths—its joys reverberate to a music that will sound through the long years of a lifetime. One of the reasons that it touches you so deeply is that it opens you up physically and emotionally. There exist parts of the human soul that can only be accessed and understood through the greatness of vulnerability.

IN MY FIRST LABOR EXPERIENCE, *my midwives kept telling me to open up. I didn't know what they meant until after the delivery of my son and my soul was cracked open. The winds of love were flowing through the open windows of my soul. It was an experience of vulnerability and freedom.*

This openness is demonstrated in labor when you reach deep inside and access your capacity to manifest the extraordinary. Intense pain and effort can be doorways to a part of yourself where you are capable of far more than you had ever dreamed possible or previously experienced. This is not a place from which you live your ordinary life. You may find it in response to the extreme needs of a situation. Birth is not the only event that may require an extraordinary response. Sometimes, we choose to bring these experiences into our lives, (as illustrated in the following example) and, sometimes, life just brings them to us. Existing in this place inside yourself takes great courage, determination, and superhuman effort. You usually only manifest these kinds of efforts for short times—most of us are not capable of sustaining the extraordinary for longer. Some people live a lifetime and never discover this place in themselves.

AN ULTRAMARATHON IS A JOURNEY *that requires dedication of one's body, mind, and soul. I usually run ultras that are between thirty-one to thirty-five miles—a long time to be on your feet in rugged terrain. A good training program builds up your body and your mind's endurance for the endeavor. The soul is what you encounter when you are on your journey.*

*I dedicate each ultra I run to honor a person in my life who has impacted and inspired me. When my mind or body tires during the race or if my soul needs refreshing, I think of the challenges they met and conquered during their lifetimes, and that inspires me to go beyond my normal limits.*

*My first ultra was in memory of a friend, Peter, who died at age eighty of complications caused by adult-onset diabetes. He never complained of the limitations of the disease, even when he gradually lost the use of his legs and then his sight. He especially never lost his smile, which could fill up a room. When my legs complained on the steep hills of that first ultra, I thought of Peter and his smile. My aches and pains felt trivial and paled when I contemplated how he embraced and overcame his everyday challenges. I ascended that hill and completed the rest of the course with a smile on my face.*

*I dedicated my second ultra to my father, who died when I was twelve. I was on my final training run when a yellow-striped snake slithered across the trail in front of me. I had never seen a snake in that area, especially a yellow-striped one. After the run, I went to see my favorite body worker. Ironically, he had placed a yellow sheet on the massage table, instead of the normal white one. When I told him of my encounter with the yellow-striped snake, he reminded me of an important aspect of snakes, which is that they shed their skins. He suggested there could be unfinished business with my father and the race might provide an opportunity to complete that loop.*

*The ultra racecourse was difficult. Seven hills, each a thousand feet of elevation gain and loss. I was on the seventh and final hill when my body shut down. I had started up the hill with determination, one foot at a time. I was absorbed, watching beads of sweat drip from my face perpendicularly to the ground, my head bent. Unconsciously, a shock wave of disbelief shot through my body when my right leg, in the process of lifting up and moving forward, instead dropped back down to the ground, stopping. I was electrified with the knowledge that I had become a silent, hollow corpse whose soul had no will to move. A statue in the middle of the trail.*

*In that moment of deep silence a voice boomed out of the deep abyss. The voice spoke, calling me by name, commanding me to "... get going ... get going now ... " I responded. I picked up my right leg and moved forward. I looked up. A fellow runner further up the trail was wearing a yellow windbreaker. I glued my eyes to that yellow windbreaker. My pace increased; soul replenished, body rejuvenated. I caught up with him. He looked at me and told me what a great job*

*I was doing. I smiled and thanked him, acknowledging his great effort also. At the summit of the hill, race volunteers cheered and told me I was almost there. Just a couple miles down the hill to the finish, they said. They were wrong. I had already completed my journey. My tears of sweat were replaced with tears of joy as I was filled with the realization that my father would have been proud, very proud, of what I had become. A cycle was complete. A skin had been shed.*

Pain is one of the greatest teachers of life. Coping with pain is the opposite of running away from it. Move into the middle of the pain. Open yourself to it. Honor what it can teach you about yourself. This is on a different level than tolerating it, enduring it. Pain's intensity can lead you to share in its power and strength. Who are we to dare to be so powerful? We are the women who birth the human beings into life on this planet. Carrying this power is a responsibility sacred to women. It frightens us. It intimidates us. It exhausts us; and, at the same time, it gives us the opportunity to be part of the energy that causes plants to grow in the spring, rivers to flow to the oceans, babies to seek their mother's milk for nourishment. It is life energy.

Another way in which birth often presents you with lessons in self-growth is in its potential to reveal the unexpected. When you are used to getting your own way, you can waste energy into trying to keep control over what happens during the birth of your baby. If birth sends you an unforeseen complication, instead of feeling helpless and defeated, you can learn about your inner strength through adaptability and acceptance. You can rise to the occasion instead of being knocked down by it. *Happiness* comes when you get what you want in life. You experience *serenity* when you want what you get. Understanding this difference between happiness and serenity, can aid in setting goals and finding value in the end result.

✦

As much as I try not to, *it has been impossible to not compare my second son's birth to my first delivery and postpartum experience. I strongly feel that a lot of my positive experience this time around is due to the deep love and commitment I have for my first son. I owe him a huge acknowledgement... for choosing to be my firstborn. His mama has learned so much already. Thanks to him, I am far further along on the path of finding my truest self. Yes, in a lot of ways, I felt defeated and like a failure from his birth and through my first year as a mother. The hilarious and unique beauty of my first son amazes me, as well as the deep, deep lessons I have learned from the insecurity, fear, questioning, and depression that I experienced. The kid is amazing. Yes, I lose my cool at times and cannot fathom why: when asked not to rub his hummus-covered hands on the side of the fridge he must do just that. But overall I'm amused, amazed, and humbled by him. I did not "fail" first time around. I was scared and lost and self-deprecating for sure. And that is simply part of the awesome journey. There is no getting it "wrong." The truth of it is, I birthed both boys in natural, beautiful, and powerful ways. Each experience has been exactly what I needed. My first year of motherhood challenged my personal identity and my need to be "perfect:" in control, to be approved of, to be liked, and to be popular. And, thank God...I have found a quieter and stronger "mama place" from which I now dream, create, grow, mother, and try to live each day. I have been supported, have asked for support, and have received it—in awesome and open ways. Yes, I am pushed by some classic toddler-testing of boundaries. Yes, the tears of exhaustion and fear have surfaced more than once. Yes, I wonder at times if I'll truly be able to "hold it together" and not dip back into depression. But mostly, it's all plain good. I am confident that the hard parts are just that, parts, and even the crazy nighttime schedule also will pass. Corny but true... the good stuff's not easy.*

How can you find a gift in *not* getting what you want from your birth experience? What can be positive about having an unexpected cesarean delivery or an induction of labor that ends up being complicated and full of medical interventions? The emotional pain around the loss of the peaceful, natural birth that you might have imagined is real and undeniable. It needs to be experienced and honored in the same way that we would process any other grief. The problem is that many women get stuck in the loss and never find their way through to the gift. In contrast, I have known several inspirational women who embraced their undesired birth journey and forged through the disappointment to create acceptance, flexibility, and gratitude. I watched them become stronger, wiser, and more mature women.

Most of us need to work on how to move forward in our lives in a healthy way after we don't get what we want. As a mother, one of the greatest functions that may be asked of you is to be the support and guidance for your children when life doesn't bring what they expected. These events may range from striking out in the baseball game to surviving the rejection of a divorce. You could experience the pain of watching your daughter miscarry a baby she spent years trying to conceive. The more that you have responded to unexpected and undesired events in your life with courage, grace, and adaptability, the more you will have empathy and wisdom to give to your children.

They learn from our experiences. If your children hear their own birth stories, including the choices you made to do what was *needed* rather than what you *wanted*; it may inspire them to live bravely and honestly. Perhaps when they themselves face unexpected or undesired circumstances, they may choose to not retreat into a sense of failure or resentment. In this way, every extra effort that you make in labor that is beyond what you ever thought would be asked of you can be dedicated to the transformation of becoming the mother your children need you to be.

*Every extra effort you make in labor can be dedicated to the transformation of becoming the mother your children need you to be.*

Guidelines for the spiritual aspect of birthing may come from the teachings of a religion or a spiritual practice. If either of these are part of your life, they can be valuable assets to help you make your inner journey through birthing and into parenthood. Practices such as prayers, meditation, or mantras can be very effective in keeping you grounded and focused through labor. Some women with a belief in God or spiritual evolvement see the process of birthing their baby as a service to something higher than themselves. This is a powerful motivator to keep going when you are tempted to give up. Belief that you are not alone and that your prayers will be heard and answered can be a great solace to a laboring woman. In asking for help be aware of the difference between asking for the pain to go away and asking for assistance in your ability to cope with the pain.

✦

AT THE VERY END, *when it seemed I couldn't push the baby out, I asked God to come into my body and take over because I couldn't do it by myself. That helped a lot, I think.*

✦

I DELIVERED MY BABIES IN THE 1950s. *It was an era when women were put to sleep for their labors. I had seen my sister birth her baby naturally and I decided that was the way I wanted to do it. When my time came, my husband wasn't allowed to stay with me and I was left to labor all alone. I turned to my faith for help and the prayer came to me, "All for Thee, most Sacred Heart of Jesus." Through hours of contractions, I repeated these words with unbroken rhythm. They were my guide, my lifeline.*

If you don't have a belief in a higher being or plan, guidelines for birth as a journey of personal growth can also be gathered from many other sources in life. Using your conscience, you can choose what is right and useful for you.

When you approach birth and parenting with an open heart, a willing mind, and pure intent you can utilize whatever happens as a pathway to becoming a better human being. This is not dependent on the external events of your baby's birth. It happens inside you. You don't even have to know how to make it happen. Just take the next step and do it to the best of your ability. A simple definition of a spiritual path is any effort to live your life from your highest, best parts. Your progress may be slow, it may seem imperceptible, but, with patient repetition, you move closer to who you wish to be. The following are some examples of spiritual aims that may be useful guideposts through the journey of birthing and parenthood.

- ❖ The wish to know who you really are and the purpose for which you are alive.

- ❖ The willingness to seek the truth instead of the comfortable illusions with which you surround yourself.

- ❖ The ability to see the beauty in the reality of life.

- ❖ The gift of experiencing inner serenity in the midst of external chaos and trauma.

- ❖ The capacity to experience love for yourself and all that surrounds you.

- ❖ The courage to live your life in a way that prepares you to die without regret.

- ❖ The cultivation of the wisdom to value that which brings meaning to your existence.

- ❖ The commitment to be present to whatever life brings you.

力

# The Value of the Birthing Experience

*The effort of the journey is connected
to the view at the end.*

If you are considering natural birth you may be faced with questions such as, "Why would you want to experience all that pain and effort when you could be comfortable?" "What's the point?" "What if something goes wrong and you need help?" The answers to these questions may lie in exploring what is important to you about birth. Throughout your life you may have been influenced from several directions in the formation of the beliefs and attitudes that affect how you value the experience of birth. This chapter begins by exploring possible sources of those influences. Then it moves into clarifying for yourself: "What are you using to measure what you value?" "Where does empowerment fit into birth?" These are the first steps in assisting you to make more intentional choices in your birthing experience. When you clarify what you value, you create guidelines for your life.

It can be helpful to ask yourself whose perspective on birthing has been important in providing a picture of what birth is about and what the experience is like. Some women find that they haven't encountered much discussion about birth. Their only exposure may have been through the public media with television, movies, the Internet, and reading material. Other women may have grown up being told the stories of their mothers' births or heard about the experiences of their sisters' or friends'. There is also the group of women who have been exposed to birth through working in a maternity care environment and face the challenge of identifying themselves as the pregnant woman instead of the provider.

✦

I GREW UP LEARNING AND BELIEVING *that birth is a normal part of womanhood (if the woman wants children, that is). My mother was very open about her experiences of having one child in a hospital and two at home. Every year on our birthdays, we were told our birth stories and the stories of how we were named. What reached me the most was the joy of each experience—even with the pain that came— and how happy she was to meet us all. The stories helped me believe that birth was an exciting event, and I always looked forward to birthing my children. As a young child, I also thought that if my mom did it, then I could do it, too, because I wanted to be just like her!*

✦

I GREW UP FEELING *very removed from the birthing process.* I only knew that my mother *had me in a hospital on twilight sleep and when she woke up she had a baby.*

*My first real understanding of birth happened in a ninth grade sex ed class where we watched a film about childbirth. It was one of those ones that, in retrospect, were meant to discourage premarital sex. After almost fainting, I decided childbirth was not for me! Too much blood and pain!*

## Societal Attitudes About Birth

We live in a society that generally does not value pain and effort. We are surrounded by advertising for products that make life easier. The more technology we create, the more we value efficiency, safety, and free time to relax. We live with the illusion that somewhere out there is the "good life," where we never lift a finger and experience only pleasure.

Nobody ever won a medal for continuing on through a long, hard labor and adding another human life to this planet. This kind of effort is applauded in only a few aspects of life: for example, working hard to advance your education or career, losing weight, or participating in sports activities. Watching athletes compete in the Olympic Games, we can't fail to appreciate the pain and effort it took to get them to where they are. Between aching and injured body parts and sheer determination to persevere, they become our societal heroes. We award them medals and put their pictures in our magazines. Women are discouraged from fully participating in natural childbirth because "it hurts too much." Train for a marathon if you want accolades for sweating and pushing through the pain.

In general, the public media, especially television, movies, and fictional books, have conveyed a message that the two most important aspects of the birth experience are that it is unbearably painful and that women must frequently be rescued by medical experts and technology from the dangerous complications that threaten moms and babies. While the over dramatization may make for exciting stories, some of us in the birthing profession are concerned that women are led to fear birth and mistrust their own capabilities of participating in this natural bodily function. When was the last time you saw television present a calm, peaceful birth that was accomplished without complications or technological intervention? The heroes of television birth stories are the doctors and nurses who save the day. The real heroes in life are the women who serve their babies by allowing them to pass through their bodies and begin their own journeys into the world.

*The real heroes in life are the women who serve their babies by allowing them to pass through their bodies and begin their own journeys into the world.*

Another place that women turn to when they are formulating their own picture of birth are books, magazines and the Internet. There is a wide range of attitudes and beliefs that are found in these sources. Many include a variety of birth stories about other women's experiences.

Some clearly support natural birth as a "womanly" activity, while others are about providing information on how to prepare for a medicalized birth. When reading this material it is useful to be aware of the degree of the author's bias when expressing her/his perspective. It is challenging to avoid the message that there is a right or wrong way to birth a baby. One of my efforts in writing this book is to help women search inside themselves for at least some of the direction in making choices concerning their own birthing experiences.

Many women turn to family and friends to form a picture of what birthing is like. Some children are raised being told their birth story over and over. Others never hear a word about it until they get closer to being parents themselves, and then have to make the effort to uncover the parts of the story that they piece together. The stories can be very supportive of women's ability to give birth or they may be passed on as tales of horrible suffering that dragged on for hours. We find some women who were frightened as children and others who were encouraged to look forward to the day when they might experience the wonder and joy of birthing. Mothers, sisters, or friends were often the storytellers. Since we tend to have close relationships with these women, their messages can have profound influences. One of the shortcomings of this method of gathering information is that it may present a rather narrow sampling of what can happen during birthing and how women choose to cope. If a sister planned a natural birth and she ended up choosing an epidural in labor, the story is often presented as, "Labor pain was so intense that any sane person would have realized it was too much and asked for an epidural, just like I did." Often part of the story includes a strong effort to convince a pregnant woman that she will need an epidural, also. It is sometimes difficult to separate the storyteller's well-wishing of others from her need to validate that she made the right choice herself. As a midwife, I wish that all women could experience the freedom to choose and receive support, laboring in whatever way works best for them.

MY MOTHER EXPERIENCED *a very traumatic birth with my older sister; something she frequently mentions, especially when angry with us. Though both of her labors were medicated, they were long and lonely—my father was the traditional "I'll wait outside" type. My mother is also an evangelical Christian, and they believe that the pain and suffering of labor is the price that women pay for Eve's acceptance of the serpent's temptation, which led to the expulsion of Adam and Eve from the Garden of Eden. As loopy as this sounds to me now, I grew up dreading childbirth.*

✦

GROWING UP, I ALWAYS HAD THE IMPRESSION THAT CHILDBIRTH *was no big deal. Six of my nine siblings were born at home and several of them had no attending midwife or doctor of any kind. I grew up in the house where I was born and thought this was how everyone did it. When my mother was in early labor she boiled shoelaces and scissors to tie off and cut the umbilical cord. She also never complained or mentioned pain in regards to her labors.*

Often women rely on their health care providers to inform them of what to expect in labor and what is most important. They might assume that the people who work in the profession of caring for new moms and babies are the experts whose opinions should be considered valid. Remember that most people in this role have spent years developing their own perspectives on birthing. When choosing your birth attendant, childbirth educator, and support people, it's beneficial to explore what their beliefs, attitudes, and philosophies are and whether they are compatible with your own. Are you interested in utilizing your inner resources when making choices and participating in the effort of birthing? Or, do you feel more comfortable relying on the expert's knowledge and technology to take a more dominant role in the process? Some people might be looking for a more even combination from each end of this spectrum. Sometimes when a couple is making the decision together there may be a need to compromise so that both people feel comfortable with their final birth plans. Often women don't recognize how open and vulnerable they might feel during labor. Your care providers are in a powerful position of influence, no matter how much you believe you will be in control of the process. Labor is not the time to put up a defensive front against the people caring for you. Take the time to find providers with whom who you can develop an allied birthing partnership.

✦

I REALLY WANTED TO FEEL UNENCUMBERED. *I wanted to feel free of the poking and prodding, and the beeping of medical equipment. Being on my own ground, in my home was empowering. I needed guidance and support, but not a timeline or set of rules to birth my baby. I needed to experience the fullness of my son's birth. I was born by cesarean section. My mother talks about her birth experience with fear and annoyance. She says we would have both died if we had not been in a hospital. Perhaps we would have, but knowing the cascading progression of medical interventions and the negative ways she viewed my birth, I knew I had to do it differently. I knew I needed to go back to the way women were supposed to birth; the way nature designed our bodies to function.*

## What Do We Measure to Determine Value for the Birth Experience?

When seeking to find value for the birth experience, it is helpful to question what is being measured to determine value. How you describe the birth experience effects how you value it. Traditionally, birth has been described in terms of intervention or lack of it. Then, you are faced with the question: "What are you calling an intervention?" I use the chart to the right in my birth preparation classes to help clients explore their attitudes about interventions. Strictly speaking, the only birth without

# LADDER OF INTERVENTIONS

**HOSPITAL INTERVENTIONS**
Infant Intensive Care
Cesarean Delivery
Vacuum Extractor/Forceps
Amnioinfusion (flushing the uterus with fluids)
Intra-uterine Pressure Monitor
Induction or Augmentation of Labor-Pharmaceutical
Analgesia (Pain medication)
Pharmaceutical Drugs
Internal Fetal Monitor
External Fetal Monitor

**OUT-OF-HOSPITAL AND HOSPITAL INTERVENTIONS**
Infant Suctioning or Resuscitation
Episiotomy
Perineal Repair (Stitching)
IV Hydration (IV fluids)
Some Pharmaceutical Drugs
Non-Pharmaceutical Induction/Augmentation of Labor
Amniotomy (Breaking the Bag of Waters)
Fetal Monitoring with Hand-Held Dopplar
Water Tub
Prayer
Diagnostic Tests (Ultrasound, Non-stress Test)
Screening Tests (Gestational Diabetes, Genetic)
Other Lab Work
Prenatal Education
Vitamins and Nutritional Supplements
Maternity Care Visits with a Midwife or Doctor

**OUT-OF-HOSPITAL INTERVENTIONS**
Acupuncture
Homeopathy
Herbs
Bodywork

interventions is one in which a woman births alone in her home with no preparation. Choosing a birth attendant, having lab work done, taking prenatal vitamins, or attending birth preparation classes are all interventions that most women who are planning a natural birth include in their prenatal care. By pausing to reexamine these activities, they begin to see a broader perspective about what can be viewed as "an intervention."

I have clients look at the Ladder of Interventions and ask them: "Where does natural birth end and medicalized birth start?" I have found that the term "natural birth" is often loaded with preconceptions and attitudes. I often use the term "low-intervention" birth instead. This does not mean that all births need *medical* interventions. Ideally, women choose a level of intervention ("natural" or "medical") based on the needs of their health or medical condition and their individual philosophies. An important part of birth preparation is to help clients move away from a right/wrong approach concerning interventions and instead base their use on what is needed to support the process. By fostering a flexible attitude about any kind of intervention, women are better equipped to cope if complications arise and interventions become necessary.

One way to make a distinction between natural interventions and medicalized interventions during labor is the effect they have on the locus of control in the birth process. Natural interventions, such as acupuncture or breast stimulation, temporarily influence the process but don't take over the body's natural feedback of pain, regulation of contractions, or progress towards delivery. Psychologically, you maintain the sense that your body retains control of the process. You carry the primary responsibility to provide the effort it takes to birth your baby. In contrast, medical interventions, such as pain medications, use of Pitocin to induce or control contraction patterns, or cesarean delivery, may come with the sense that they are taking over control. Your emotional and mental connection to the process changes as a medicine, machine, or an instrument directed by another person's decisions determine the course of events. While you still carry some of the responsibility, you assume a more passive role as your efforts are assisted by technology.

There are trade-offs either way in either choosing or not choosing to use interventions during the birth process. Sometimes medical needs arise that necessitate their use if your birth is not proceeding in a normal pattern. This often tips the scale when choosing whether or not to utilize interventions. For instance, using an epidural may be suggested if your labor has been progressing slowly and you haven't slept in more than a day. Allowing you to sleep and recover from your fatigue may improve the chances of delivering vaginally and avoiding cesarean delivery. However, we live in a society where we can voluntarily choose to include technology even when the birth process is proceeding normally. An example of this would be choosing to have an elective epidural when you have been laboring for ten hours and you are dilating normally. There is no need for a judgment about whether or not you decide on the epidural. Each woman must measure the value of the trade-offs for herself and decide what is best for her. Either way, it is helpful to be prepared ahead of time with a clear understanding of the challenges that may be included in each pathway.

The most common challenges for natural childbirth are usually the levels of pain and exhaustion that are encountered. There are also occasions when birth doesn't progress normally or warning signs occur that cannot be ignored. There is no guarantee that everything will go as planned; and, sometimes, interventions are necessary whether you want them or not. The payoffs of natural birth are a strong sense of accomplishment, empowerment, and self-growth.

The draw back of medicalized birth (either when it is elective or there is a medical need requiring it) is the potential for some degree of feeling disconnected from your body and losing control of the process. Additionally, the use of medical interventions may increase the chance of complications arising from the interventions themselves. The advantages may include a lessening of the experience of pain and fatigue. Medical interventions also are used to remedy or compensate for any medical condition that has complicated the birth process. In these situations, they may make birth more predictable and safe.

◆

I CHOSE NATURAL CHILDBIRTH *because it seemed like the only choice I could really put my heart into. I chose it because I was born at home, because I didn't want strangers at my birth, and because I wanted to feel comfortable and safe. Mostly I chose it because it seemed right for me—I know it doesn't feel that way for everybody.*

An example of the gifts and challenges of medicalized birth might be seen in a woman who decides to have her labor induced and get an epidural as soon as possible. If the interventions are successful, we might see the following scenario ten hours later. She's sitting up in bed, relatively comfortable, rested, and capable of conversation or napping. Since her cervix is dilating effectively in response to the Pitocin-induced contractions, she is relieved in believing that her baby will probably be born today. Since most epidurals don't leave enough sensation or strength in the legs to allow walking or standing, she has been in bed since the epidural was inserted. She cannot feel her bladder and therefore she has a urinary catheter in place to eliminate the need for urination. In order to maintain an adequate fluid volume in her body and prevent low blood pressure (which could cause problems for the baby when an epidural is in place) she has an IV in her arm dripping in fluids. An automatic blood pressure cuff on her other arm periodically inflates to monitor for low blood pressure. The Pitocin is still being run through an accessory line onto the IV. Once Pitocin is started in a labor it is not usually completely turned off because the contractions usually will stop if the synthetic hormone is not continually stimulating the contraction pattern. The amount of Pitocin being delivered into the IV can be turned up or down depending on the regularity of the contraction pattern and the baby's tolerance of the contractions. In order to monitor these two factors there are two devices strapped around her abdomen. One measures the frequency and length of the contractions. The other measures the baby's heartbeat pattern as it relates to the contraction pattern. In this way, if the contractions are too strong or frequent and effect the baby's blood flow it will usually be indicated by specific heart rate patterns. If this occurs, the Pitocin levels can be turned down or off and usually the baby's heart rate will return to a normal pattern. As she lies there she has six different lines coming off of her body either putting in medication, removing waste products, or monitoring various processes. If any complications arise, additional medications, procedures, or monitoring devices may be utilized. If she has difficulty knowing how to push and she isn't progressing she might have to experience more pain when the epidural may have to be turned down to allow her to have more sensation and, thus, be able to push more effectively. Finally, after pushing harder than she ever thought she could, her baby is laid across her chest and, in that moment, her heart feels like it will burst with joy. This is a description of a normal medicalized birth without any complications. The majority of women in this country have epidurals and many utilize Pitocin to either induce labor (start contractions) or augment labor (make the contractions stronger or more regular once they have started).

*Finally, after pushing harder than she ever thought she could, her baby is laid across her chest and, in that moment, her heart feels like it will burst with joy.*

✦

WHEN I ARRIVED AT THE HOSPITAL *I was in a lot of pain, with every contraction causing searing back pain. I got in the tub, which I was hoping was going to bring me great relief. Unfortunately, I had such incredible back pain, that I couldn't lie back and relax; instead having to sit straight up. I tried this for a bit but then felt like I wasn't getting enough relief. I tried sterile water papules injected into my back, taking a shower, sitting on a birth ball, moving around. When the sterile water injection relief wore off, my back pain returned with a vengeance. I tried massage and the birth ball again but as my contractions became increasingly closer together, I began to feel myself losing my ability to cope. I was contracting every 1-2 minutes, couldn't empty my bladder, and really was beginning to question whether I could tolerate labor for much longer. I asked for sterile water injections again, but this time I didn't get as much relief. I was now 6cm dilated and while I was making progress, I was still aware of the fact that it was taking me a while, and that I still had a lot further to go. I decided at this point that I wanted an epidural; I couldn't bear the thought of feeling that much pain for many more hours.*

*My birth team helped me accept my request for pain medicine. I felt like it was okay for me to "give in." Once I made the decision to accept pain relief medications, it became increasingly difficult to cope. I had to wait for an IV to be placed, and at least some IV fluids to infuse. After the epidural was in place, I rested and my husband fell asleep. It was strange to be in labor but not feel pain. However, I was immensely happy to not be feeling the pain any longer.*

*I had hoped to avoid pain medications, but when it came down to it, I realized that wasn't what was important to me. My faith in my body to do its job had been shaken when we had a hard time getting pregnant. What I had desired from my birth was an experience that would restore that faith. I got that!*

An example of the gifts and challenges of natural birth might be seen in the following scenario. A woman has chosen to birth with a low use of interventions. She has had her patience tried as she waited ten days past her due date and dealt with repeated calls from family and friends asking if she has had the baby yet. This morning at 10 a.m. she had acupuncture induction to encourage her body to begin the labor process. Four hours later, at 2 p.m., contractions began. It is now 4 a.m. the next morning, she is 6 cm dilated and she has been in active labor for two hours. Since she didn't sleep well last night, she is beginning to feel exhausted. The contractions already hurt more than she thought they would. She is concerned that the stronger contractions that are probably ahead of her, combined with her fatigue, may be overwhelming. She has no idea how much longer she'll have to continue with this process. While the water birth tub is helpful, it doesn't provide as much relief as she had counted on. Her moans during contractions start to take on a sharp-edged pitch. She opens her eyes to find her midwife at her side. Her midwife asks her how she is feeling. She speaks honestly about her doubts; not sure if she made the right choice about birthing naturally. Her midwife validates that what is being asked of her is a great effort and affirms all that it has taken to get this far. The midwife also affirms her confidence that the birthing process is unfolding quite normally and reassures her that she has the capability to continue on the journey. Suggestions are made to the laboring woman to dig deep and open to places in herself that may be unknown to her: greater levels of endurance, more allowing of stronger pain sensations, deeper trust in the freedom of open vulnerability. The midwife assures her that she is surrounded by loving support and acknowledges that no one else can do it for her. The laboring woman chooses to continue. She encounters even stronger contractions and even greater fatigue. She loses track of time, focusing on just getting through each contraction as it

*Looking down into his eyes for the first time is a moment she'll never forget.*

comes. After hours of such effort, she begins to feel the need to have a bowel movement. She tells her midwife, who then does a vaginal exam, and explains that she is feeling the baby's head dropping deeply into her vagina and past the cervical opening. The urge to bring her baby into the world becomes even more important than the pain of the contractions. Her pushing efforts begin and two hours later her arms reach out to receive her warm, wet baby. Looking down into his eyes for the first time is a moment she'll never forget.

✦

IN SOME WAYS, I FEEL THAT BIRTHING MY SECOND BABY *hurt more than my first because I didn't run away energetically or emotionally from the experience in the same way. I left the judging at the back door and actually felt what was going on, as it happened... After awhile, I could actually feel his head in the birth canal. I could feel my vagina open and I could most definitely feel that "ring of fire." I felt my baby be born. I felt myself deliver the little guy. I was there, aware, alive, present. HE was there, alive and present. I felt like a competent, responsible, committed, and whole-hearted participant. I did it. I birthed my baby boy. I loved feeling his head at last come through and then his body, sort of squiggly after the head. I felt completely there when I took him into my arms for the first time. I felt in love as I looked down at him. I felt like a success. I felt grounded, successful, and present. I felt capable, relieved, and in love. And I felt*

*healed from much of the powerless self-deprecation, judgment, and*
*expectations I had heaped on myself first time around. My son was*
*here... I was here; fully and completely. How grateful I am.*

# Empowered Birthing

Restricting our description of birthing to what interventions are used leaves out a major part of what birth means to us as mothers and women. Instead, when we describe birth as it relates to a woman's inner experience, a different perspective and value emerges. The possibility arises of empowered birthing in which you use your own inner resources to face the challenges of birth. As an empowered woman, you commit to full participation whether or not you choose interventions or they become necessary for medical reasons. In this way, the birth process provides an opportunity for your transformation and maturation. Your inner journey of self-growth parallels your baby's entry into the world. In viewing birth from this perspective a powerful value for full participation in the birthing experience is revealed. The beauty and strength of empowered birthing is that any interventions that might be necessary, whether they are natural or medicalized, are much less important. The focus instead is on your own inner knowing that you have served the process to the best of your ability. Your transformation into motherhood enriches you as a woman and as a human being. Valuing participation in the birth process in this way has the potential to build a strong and clear motivation that may carry you through when you face the challenges of labor.

*The possibility arises of empowered birthing in which you use your own inner resources to face the challenges of birth.*

An analogy can be made with three hikers setting off to climb a steep mountain because they've heard that the view from the top is spectacular. They've put everything in their backpacks that they think they'll need and hoist them onto their shoulders. As the hours pass, the sun gets hotter and the packs feel heavier. More hours go by and the path is much steeper with less shade. Everyone's shoulders are telling them that next time it might be advisable to pack lighter. Oh, and did I mention the blisters from the new hiking boots? A helicopter suddenly arrives on the scene and spots the hikers. Using a loud speaker (because helicopters make a lot of noise on a quiet mountain side) they ask if anyone would like a ride to the top. One of the hikers decides that she's had enough adventuring and indicates that she'll take them up on the offer. They drop down a ladder and up she goes. (like that wouldn't be an adventure in itself!).

The helicopter speeds away and leaves the other two hikers to continue the uphill climb. More hours pass and it's not getting any easier. Now the path is rocky and they are pulling themselves over boulders. Finally, a rock gives way under one of the hikers and she falls, breaking her ankle. Clearly, she's not going to make it to the top on her own two feet. No one is to blame. Her plan to climb a mountain just got diverted into dealing with her injury. As the hikers are considering how to get her off the mountainside, the helicopter swings back by on its homeward bound trip. The hikers wave it down and make it clear that they need help. This time the helicopter staff lower a hammock and, with a bit of maneuvering, manage to rescue her and speed her off to the nearest emergency room.

The final hiker takes a long breath and decides that she's just too close to give up now. She digs deep and finds she has enough stamina left to push on. Alone on the mountain, all she has to rely on is herself. It's quiet up that high and her relationship to the world somehow seems different. She's never been this far from another human being. She's never been this tired or this sore. It takes more than just her body to move forward. Something inside her has to stay focused on affirming her choice with every step she takes. Finally, she arrives at the top of the mountain ridge and there is enough light left to see why she was told the view would be spectacular. Sitting on a warm rock, she takes it in. The panorama is the same as what the riders in the helicopter saw but her experience of what she sees is different. The effort of the journey is connected to the view at the end.

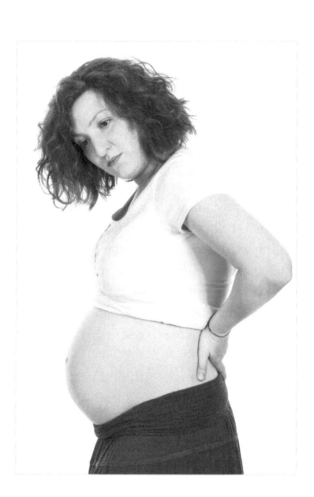

力

# Courage

*May your love for your baby motivate you
to face your own dragons.*

Some women find that, right along with the joy (or sometimes surprise) of finding out they are pregnant, comes an unexpected increase in worries, anxieties, and fears. This vague sense of insecurity about what life will bring may continually arise throughout pregnancy, birth, and parenting. Even though most pregnant women have never seen themselves as worriers, many wonder what is wrong with them now. This increased anxiety is a subconscious signal that a major change is underway and your life is about to undertake a 180-degree turn. Thus begins a journey of transitions through pregnancy, birth, and on into the many stages of parenting.

✦

MANY TIMES IN THE LAST EIGHT MONTHS *I have heard, "Oh, it's your second baby; you know what to expect. You've done it all before, you'll be fine." What I've been discovering over the course of this second pregnancy is that, no, I don't know what to expect. And, no, I haven't done this before. Not with this baby and not at this time.*

*When I was told that this baby was breech at thirty-four weeks a tremendous amount of anxiety started to resurface in me that I had been suppressing throughout this pregnancy. There was so much emotion that came bubbling out of me. As I thought about it, I wondered if it was because of the baby that I had miscarried the year before. I still had a fear of losing this baby, too, and every little difference this time sent me into that vulnerable place that was so raw since my miscarriage. I hadn't done this before. I hadn't navigated the emotions of carrying a second baby with new worries. My first baby had been at a time in my life when I was blissfully naïve and innocent. I hadn't known how to love so deeply and feel so completely before my daughter taught me how; and now I knew the pain of losing that love from my subsequent miscarriage and feared it could happen again. I had lost my trust in the process unfolding as it should.*

*I now had to fight my fears at every turn in this pregnancy. As my feet started to swell, when they hadn't before, I worried. When I had pains in my ribs, when I hadn't before, I worried. When I learned my baby was breech, I really worried. When I tested positive for Group B Strep, I again began to worry that something would go wrong and I wouldn't be able to birth this baby as I had my daughter. As I felt myself spiraling out of control in all this worry I realized my baby was trying to communicate with me that we were on a new journey and that this little spirit had its own gifts to teach us and I hadn't been listening. As the inevitable birth neared, I knew I needed to do some inward work to make my hopes for a natural home birth a reality. I realized that in comparing my three pregnancies, I was letting fear guide me. I needed to embrace this pregnancy as its own unique experience. I had to listen and walk down this path in full surrender, knowing that my body and baby knew what to do. I had to find a way to be in the innocence of this experience and accept what may come because that is when I am my strongest, bravest, and most loving: when I am in the moment.*

Bringing a baby into your life cannot help but have a profound effect on how you will experience each and every day. Once you are a parent, you will live your life with a part of you always aware of your child's presence in the world. Your familiar life is giving way to a great new adventure. No matter how much you prepare, you can't get around the unknowns that will line up before you concerning the upcoming birth and your life beyond that. It is normal to have ideas and plans about what the end results may be. It is also true that pregnancy and the birth of your child include the inherent possibility that things

*Once you are a parent, you will live your life with a part of you always aware of your child's presence in the world.*

may not turn out the way you anticipate or want. The ability to face your fears and stay present in reality can be a focus of inner work during pregnancy, birth, and parenting.

◆

I HAD/HAVE A LOT MORE FEARS AND WORRIES *about parenting than I did about pregnancy and childbirth. I feel like there is so much more room to mess up when it comes to being a parent. I've been afraid at different times of getting angry, wanting to get away, and just wondering if I'm cut out to care for another human being. Part of the fear/pain for me is thinking no one else deals with these emotions.*

## From the Familiar into the Unknown

When you closely observe the experience of fear you may discover that it presents itself when the possibility of an unwanted outcome is perceived. Fear is a warning sign that danger might be lurking, alerting you to pay attention and try to avoid it. As long as the imagined threat remains a possibility, fear continues to get your attention by making you uncomfortable. In the instances when the undesired event actually occurs and the escape options for a more desirable outcome are gone, fear doesn't have a purpose anymore and leaves you alone. This is illustrated in the reports from people who have survived serious auto accidents, such as driving off cliffs. When they first lose control of the car they may feel immobilized with fear as they are skidding towards the edge of the road. Once it becomes clear that, indeed, they are going over the edge, people later report that time seems to stretch out and they have a sense of peacefully being there in the present moment. *Fear is about what could happen; not what is happening.*

◆

WE WERE DRIVING DOWN THE ROAD *just after a quick rain shower. There were five of us in the car, none of us old enough to drive. The boys in the back kept egging on the driver to speed up before we got caught. Easily influenced as most of us are at that time in our lives, she sped up to sixty miles per hour on a winding and slick country road. I tried not to lose my cool (after all there were boys in the back) but I felt real fear taking over. I quickly put on my seat belt and asked her to slow down. There was so much yelling to speed up from the back of the car it was useless. The next thing I remember is flying. It felt like I was fifty feet in the air. Everything went silent. I knew that I was about to die. There was nothing that I could do except be quiet and still. I had to completely let go of even trying to fight because my fate was so obvious. I had to just be in that moment, surrendering completely. Although I remember thinking for a moment, "I am too young for this to happen," there was this feeling of peace that settled and overrode that thought. In my greatest moment of fear, I found my greatest moment of clarity and peace. Although I am sure it was only seconds, I saw before me all of my happiest moments of my life in slow motion. Letting go of my fear brought me this moment of great happiness. I was weightless and free of fear. When our car-turned-airplane finally met up with a tree; this moment stopped and the blood-curdling screaming began, along with the smashing of my bones.*

Many of the biggest fears concerning childbirth are about the unknown. If we could just tell you how much the contractions will hurt, how long labor will last, whether or not there will be a problem for the baby, then you would know what will be required of you and you could prepare yourself. I have worked with many pregnant women who have previously run marathons. They have pointed out that, while they know they are capable of perseverance, when they are running they always know how much farther they have to go. Labor doesn't provide such clear mileposts.

## The Medical World's Relationship to Risk

One of the goals of modern technology is to improve maternity care by making pregnancy and birth more predictable and safer. We have developed screening tests for fetal developmental problems, monitors for continual assessment of the baby's heart pattern in labor, Pitocin induction to know when labor will start, and elective cesarean births to know exactly when a baby will be born. The challenge comes in walking the line between utilizing modern maternity care and trusting the birthing process. The use of interventions can be appropriately indicated by medical complications. When they are utilized only to have increased control of a normal pregnancy or labor they can potentially decrease a woman's sense of participation and belief in her own capability to birth her baby. Some women respond to their maternity care with increased feelings of anxiety about the potential risks for their baby and their pregnancy. It has raised doubts for them that their labors will precede normally or that their bodies can be relied upon to evade the possible complications of delivery. This is certainly not the intent of maternity care providers when they order screening tests or quote statistical risks to their patients.

✦

> I THINK THE MOST DIFFICULT PART *of having gestational diabetes for me was the fact that my physiology—upon which I was relying completely in this process—was malfunctioning. Because I was approaching birth from the standpoint that as long as I trusted, things would happen as they needed to, I was disproportionately disturbed that something was amiss.*

The last few decades of medicine have been permeated with the concept of evidence-based practice and management decisions based on risk assessment. The impetus for this was an effort to improve patient care by conducting sound research on the methods we use to provide our medical services. Then we can change our practices to provide the best care we can. For example, we have investigated what the best techniques are for a procedure, which medicines are most effective, and what are the best tools to diagnose and monitor a pathological condition. As a result of research two areas have been expanded in maternity care that have strongly influenced the role risk plays in how providers practice.

The first advancement is our improved ability to predict the risk factors that are associated with the complications of pregnancy and birth. This means we have figured out how to recognize some of the warning signs that show a person has a significantly greater chance of developing a problem in the future than someone who doesn't present the same picture. It doesn't mean that she will develop the condition, only that she is at greater risk for it. Most of the time women with elevated risk factors go on to have healthy pregnancies. Only a small percentage will have significant complications. Once research has confirmed the statistical presence of these risk factors, we are then faced with the question of what to do with the information. In an effort to assist people in making informed choices about their health care, part of prenatal care is focused on educating patients about their risk factors. This includes discussions about their statistical risk of complications, further testing that might clarify if they truly have a pathological diagnosis, and possible interventions that might decrease their chances of an undesirable outcome.

> *Most of the time women with elevated risk factors go on to have healthy pregnancies.*

The second area of development that has influenced the prediction of maternity risk has been the utilization of more screening tests for our normal, healthy pregnant women. Most prenatal care includes at least one ultrasound during the pregnancy and the offer of genetic screening (ultrasounds and lab tests to determine a baby's risk of having different abnormal conditions). For these and other routine tests done during a pregnancy, it's important to distinguish between a *screening* test and a *diagnostic* test. The results from a screening test come back as a percentage of each woman's specific risk of carrying a baby with a specific abnormality. For example, a pregnant woman decides to do genetic screening for some of the possible chromosomal abnormalities. At twelve weeks of pregnancy she has a screening ultrasound and a blood draw. She waits a week and the test results come back indicating that she has a one in one hundred fifty chance of delivering a baby with Down syndrome. That means that if there were one hundred fifty pregnant women with identical results, statistically, one hundred forty nine of them would have normal babies and one would have Down syndrome. Because her risk is higher than that of the normal population, she is offered a diagnostic test called an amniocentesis. The diagnostic test will give her a definite yes or no as to whether or not her baby has Down syndrome. If she decides to not have the diagnostic test she will continue her pregnancy with the knowledge that "her risk is higher than that of the normal population." Some women who chose not to continue with diagnostic testing report back that they feel so disturbed about their pregnancy that they wish they had never done the screening test in the first place. Because of this, it seems advisable that if a woman decides to do the screening test, she needs to be prepared to go on for diagnostic testing if the results come back as increased risk. If she has the diagnostic test she usually has a very good chance (in the above example it would be greater than ninety-nine per cent) that the results will be reassuring,

*The dance continues between utilizing technology to predict the chance of risk and supporting a woman's confidence in her body and ability to birth.*

although it may take one to two weeks of waiting to get those results. The problem is that some women whose amniocentesis results come back normal still describe feeling that their confidence in their body has been undermined by the whole experience.

The dance continues between utilizing technology to predict the chance of risk and supporting a woman's confidence in her body and ability to birth. It's not a black and white picture. On the positive side, technology has increased our ability to detect medical conditions for moms or unborn babies who aren't showing symptoms of a problem. If we have a diagnosis we can begin treatment earlier, or at least be prepared sooner for a concerning situation. This may improve the chances of a better outcome. For those clients who have negative screens they are generally reassured.

Besides the impact on maternal self-confidence and peace of mind, there are other consequences from increased screening and management decisions based on risk factors. One of the most influential results is the increase in medical interventions for diagnoses that, in themselves, do not cause long-term damage to the baby or mother, but are associated with increased risks of conditions that could cause permanent undesired outcomes. An example of this is the increase in inductions of labor. Five of the most common reasons for induction are prolonged pregnancies, diet-controlled gestational diabetes, gestational hypertension (elevated blood pressures with no other symptoms), low levels of the fluid that surrounds the baby inside the uterus, and advanced maternal age (thirty-five years and beyond). None of these conditions necessarily cause damage unless they proceed to a more complicated diagnosis. The reasoning behind starting labor artificially is to get the baby delivered before there is a chance of the potentially damaging complication occurring. The positive result of inductions is that the small percentage of babies who statistically would have developed the complication usually have better outcomes. The majority of the other women who statistically would have had healthy babies receive increased medical intervention, even if their intent was to avoid it. The difficulty lies in the reality that we have not yet developed the capability to predict which babies will have the complication and which will be born in a healthy state.

The answer to this situation is not simple. From the provider's point of view they are offering the safest care they can, in the belief that this is what people want and will feel reassured by their efforts. This is true for some people. Other people respond by feeling that there is too much focus on what could go wrong and not enough on affirming that the pregnancy process and delivery is proceeding normally. Another significant influence comes from the risk management departments of hospitals. One of their jobs is to help prevent medical malpractice suits from being settled against the institutions and the healthcare providers. They put strong pressure on providers to insure that patients are informed of the risks in any medical situation. If a lawsuit is filed, informed patients have a more difficult time claiming that they didn't know there could be a complication.

In a perfect world we would replace the screening tests and risk factors with simple, economical diagnostic tests. We haven't developed the technology yet to do that. Working with what we have is getting us closer to that ideal, but there is a long way to go. In the meantime, providers need to be more aware of the anxiety that they are creating when they discuss risk. Pregnant couples need to work at responding to the news that there is an increased risk of a complication with less emotional magnification and more focus on the chances of a normal baby and pregnancy. Remember that a statistical risk of one in one hundred gives a ninety-nine percent chance of a healthy baby.

## Predictability and the Unknown

Not only is birthing full of unknowns, but, particularly for first time moms, the whole process is unfamiliar. Birthing usually happens only a few times in a woman's life. Therefore, most women aren't likely to approach the experience with feelings of familiarity. Also, the culture of birth in this country adds to our fears. No matter how much you read or hear stories about birthing, your final reassurance that you can do it usually has to come from yourself. Remember, transformation is never free. Paying the price without knowing the cost is the way through to the other side. That is the magic of birth and the mystery of life.

*Transformation is never free. Paying the price without knowing the cost is the way through to the other side. That is the magic of birth and the mystery of life.*

◆

WHEN I WAS 29 YEARS OLD I STARTED *having dreams about having a baby, about being pregnant, about my young child. I had these dreams so often that I started to feel like I couldn't escape the thoughts about babies during the day. I realized I really wanted and felt ready for a baby. Of course I didn't have a stable relationship, job, or place to live, but the feeling persisted. I told my partner about the feeling that I was ready for a baby. I told him that if he was ready for that, I wanted to work on our relationship with the intent to get married and have children together. I remember crying as I said it because I was so scared of what I was admitting, as well as how vulnerable I felt saying it to him. He couldn't give me an answer.*

*I broke off the relationship and left on a trip for a couple weeks. When I returned he said he wanted to be together. I was not intending to get pregnant, as the relationship had not moved forward as I had hoped. Then, my great-grandmother died, a woman who had been very important to me in my childhood. During that time my cycle went from a predictable 28 days to 21 days and I conceived. I was scared but I knew that I wanted the baby. I knew that it was right that I would bring a baby into the world with my great-grandmother's passing. I felt her spirit had influenced my body. I felt immediately connected to my growing child. Even in my fear of being alone I felt an even stronger sense of rightness with the pregnancy.*

*I worried about being alone. I worried I couldn't make it financially and I would have to go to my family. I felt my family was ashamed that I was an unwed mother. It was more than a feeling. They were very clear about it. They wanted me to move home and they didn't want to support me unless I moved in with them. I felt determined to make it without them and vowed to myself that I never would ask them for money. Unfortunately, this left me more vulnerable to staying in a relationship with my child's father. I needed someone and, despite the unhealthiness of the relationship, I allowed it to continue. My choice to do that strained my friendships. They couldn't understand why I would stay in such a terrible relationship but none of them lived nearby and none of them were with me on a daily or even weekly basis. It was very painful. These struggles dominated my pregnancy. Even through those issues, I felt a deep sense that what I was doing was absolutely right. I was in awe of the process of pregnancy, what my body was doing, how amazingly powerful the bond to my child was, and she wasn't even in my arms yet! The pressures and stress escalated after my daughter was born. I did find new friendships and repaired others, but I had three extremely lonely and difficult years while I made my way.*

Recognizing that you don't live in a risk-free environment can help put some perspective on the fears that come up around birth. Reviewing your life in search of experiences when you encountered risks and survived can sometimes help you to realize you have a greater capacity for courage than your fears would have you believe. For many women our greatest courage arises when we encounter emotional risks such as opening up to the vulnerability of an intimate relationship or packing up our cars and moving cross-country. We are more courageous than we give ourselves credit for.

The relationship between fear and the unfamiliar became clear to me during a trip to Peru. I was traveling with a group along the Amazon River, taking side trips up into the rain forest. We were accompanied by an experienced guide who had grown up in one of the villages along the river. He instructed us in the many precautions that were needed to travel safely and prevent unwanted contacts with snakes, poisonous ants, etc. We wore leather gaiters around our legs, never put our foot or our hand in a place that we hadn't first looked at, and always used a flashlight when walking at night. I was particularly aware that this area was inhabited by fur-de-lances, one of the most poisonous snakes in the world. I finally had to admit to myself that I had brought a fairly significant fear about jungles with me that was irrational but still clearly present. One day he told us a story from his childhood about a time when he and his brother were out playing in the forest. They realized they were lost. As it started getting dark they decided to climb the tallest tree and look for the river to find their way home. Something inside me commented, "You couldn't pay me to climb a jungle tree in the dark, not knowing what my hand was going to encounter." Yet, he spoke of the event as though the tree climbing was the easiest part. I thought: A fur-de-lance would kill him just as fast as it would kill me. How could he be so comfortable wandering around the rain forest as a child? I asked him how he ever felt comfortable as a parent allowing his toddlers out the front door with the forest so close by. His answer was that they simply taught their children safety skills for surviving in their environment. It was really quite rare that people died of snakebites. The risks in his world were familiar to him while for me the unusual environment magnified my perception of their threat.

I don't consider myself a particularly fearful person. Why were my experiences in Peru bringing up such an awareness of the risks that

> *We are more courageous than we give ourselves credit for.*

surrounded me? Then I imagined inviting one of the river villagers to sit in the car next to me going sixty miles an hour during rush-hour traffic. Since their primary modes of transport are canoeing and walking, I suspected that they might view such a car ride with the same awareness of risk as I did about fur-de-lances. Our perception of risk is largely affected by whether or not the situation is a familiar part of our

*Our perception of risk is largely affected by whether or not the situation is a familiar part of our lives.*

lives. We are surrounded by potential danger with which we have become accustomed. We walk in city neighborhoods where we could be mugged, we bicycle on busy streets, we ski down mountains at thirty miles an hour, we take medications with potentially dangerous side effects. We know there are potential risks there and we take what precautions we can. We follow driving laws and expect others to do the same. We watch for drug reactions and change the medication at their first occurrence. These risks don't stop us from living our lives.

## Transforming Fear

Transforming your experience of fear into respect for potential danger is a useful way to work with fears and anxieties about the unknown. By shifting your perspective you recognize other possibilities and acknowledge that the potential danger is only one of the possible outcomes in a given situation. You can separate from the emotional reaction to risk and, therefore, gain a sense of balance by seeing a bigger picture. You don't ignore the danger, but neither do you give it more than its share of influence. This reckoning provides two advantages. First, while it doesn't suppress the emotion, it takes fear out of the director's seat when it comes to making choices. At that moment, your world opens and you become aware of other opportunities that were previously obscured. The potential danger is acknowledged as only a part of the information you use in coming to a decision. Secondly, respecting danger allows you to be better prepared and more calmly capable of dealing with a problem should it actually manifest. When you make a decision from a fear base, you often don't end up where you want to be.

This transformation from fear into respect may feel like more than you can pull off in the middle of coping with contractions. This is where the presence of your care-provider may assist you by bringing in the energy of confidence and guidance. A midwife's, doctor's, or nurse's years of experience have often made them familiar with birthing and the potential risks surrounding it. Hopefully, they have learned a healthy respect for what can happen without losing the perspective that most births happen just fine on their own. One of the roles of the care-provider is to hold the energy of respect with quiet surveillance and to be prepared to step in if a danger becomes real, instead of just a possibility.

I learned something about fear and receiving help when I was white-water rafting one summer. After only an hour on the river and many exciting rapids, I developed a strong trust in our river guide. He knew what he was doing and I felt confident that he was watching out for us. He announced that we were coming upon a waterfall that was not safe for rafting, and we needed to get out and portage around the falls. We followed the trail he indicated and ended up on a twenty- foot cliff overlooking the river. While we were admiring the falls that we had just passed, it started to dawn on me that the trail ended there. The boats had already been pushed over the falls and were waiting in the water below. Our guide explained that we were each going to jump into the water and then swim as hard as we could to catch up to the raft, thus avoiding being swept on down through the next rapids. There was a very specific angle we had to jump from and we had to push off hard to clear the shelf under the cliff. Now, I am not particularly fond of the sudden constriction I feel in my abdomen when I find myself free-falling through space. The thought of jumping off a 20-foot cliff into rapidly moving 40-degree water was definitely challenging. There was also no denying the risk involved if I didn't do it correctly. However, I had set out on an adventure and I wasn't about to back down. I watched two people jump off with the guide standing next to them and then stepped up before I lost my courage. As I did so the guide turned to address the rest of the group again. I waited until he was done and had turned his attention back to me. I lightly rested my hand on his, counted "one, two, three," and pushed off.

We continued on down the river and I reflected on why it was so important for me to wait until I had the guide's full attention before jumping. I didn't want to jump alone. I had plenty of voices inside me telling me to swallow my pride and find another trail down to the shore. This was crazy and what was I trying to prove anyway? But I wanted to jump. I wanted this day to be different from other days. I needed his confidence right next to me confirming that this was a wise thing to do. I trusted him enough that I chose to listen to his guidance over the frightened warnings coming from inside me. It was then that I recognized that laboring women often give their midwife, doctor, or nurse the same trust. For example, when they are feeling overwhelmed by contractions and choose to listen to their provider's guidance to let go even more, they can ride on her confidence to jump off the cliff that is challenging them.

✦

IN THE EXPERIENCE OF LABOR *there were times when I did not know how I would continue, especially before I let go of my thoughts and surrendered to my physical body. In my moments of doubt, the midwives assured me over and over again, "You know how to do this. This is what you were made for." Their belief in me helped me believe in myself.*

## Reality and Imagination

The second important piece about fear is that it only exists in imagination concerning the possibilities of a future event. During your pregnancy you may be flooded with the "what ifs." While everyone seems to have their own individual versions, there are many common themes that my pregnant women have shared with me. These might include:

**What if** something happens during the birth and my baby is not normal or dies?

**What if** my vagina or perineum tears?

**What if** I lose control of the choices about what will happen to my body?

**What if** I don't "keep it together" and make a fool of myself?

**What if** I'm just closing my eyes and not worrying enough?

**What if** I end up with interventions I don't want or a transport to a hospital?

**What if** the caregiver I trust or my support team isn't there for me when my baby comes?

**What if** I have a bowel movement in front of everyone while I'm pushing out my baby?

**What if** I "can't do it" and I end up begging for an epidural or a cesarean birth?

**What if** something goes wrong and I have to face all those people who told me I should never have tried a natural birth in the first place?

**What if** I gain too much weight and never lose it all again?

**What if** I don't like breast-feeding or being a mother?

**What if** I'm a terrible parent and I ruin my child's chances in life?

✦

I HAVE BEEN AN ATHLETE MY WHOLE LIFE—*I was a scholarship athlete in college and then did triathalons and ran a marathon after that. My body had been through a lot up until that point, and I knew what it was like to push myself physically and mentally. I'd been able to push through pain in other situations. This left me feeling pretty confident in my ability to give birth. On the other hand, I also knew the experience of giving birth was going to be like nothing else my body, or being, had ever been through; so there was still an element of fear there. What if the pain was so much more than I had ever fathomed it could be? Was I taking the whole thing too lightly? I actually started to worry that I wasn't worrying enough; and that the lack of worrying was going to leave me less prepared. In the end, I thought, "If all these other women can do it then so can I!" I let go of worrying about not worrying, knowing I was preparing by taking birth classes, reading the right books, and being well taken care of by my midwives. In the end, giving birth was unlike anything else I'd ever been through. But I went about it the same as I go about other things in life—focus and just do it! It was pretty fast and intense, but absolutely the most amazing thing I have done, or will ever do—physically, mentally, and spiritually!*

Courage is doing what is needed in the reality of the present moment instead of being immobilized by the threat of potential danger. Just as fear only exists in imagination, courage only exists in reality. The need for courage is easily conceptualized when danger actually happens and you're looking eye-to-eye with the tiger. In your daily life, rather than fear in response to danger, you are more likely to experience worry and anxiety in response to subtle risks. These can feel like nagging concerns that are often hard to name and, yet, still make you uneasy. The list of "what ifs" from above are sometimes what lie beneath the nagging worries or anxieties.

*Fear only exists in imagination concerning the possibilities of a future event.*

Having the courage to identify, recognize and/or face them can allow them their proper place as simply a possibility in the future.

The first step in freeing yourself from anxiety is to identify the beliefs that surround the "what ifs." Remember that a belief is acceptance by the mind that something is true or real. The next step comes in questioning whether the beliefs are true about something happening in reality or an imagination about a possible future. Your courage brings you the willingness and strength to push through the illusions you have accepted in order to come to the reality that lies beyond. Fear can act as a buffer, hiding a boundary that some part of you believes needs protecting. When you acknowledge inner illusion you often experience a sense of vulnerability. This may be the price of living a real life. The courage to find the truth is the doorway through the limitations with which fear imprisons you.

You may be reluctant to examine your concerns about giving birth and becoming a mother. You may believe that putting any attention or energy towards negative outcomes will draw undesired events in your direction. "If I don't acknowledge it; it doesn't exist." As a midwife, I have found that ignoring or suppressing fear does not make it go away or diminish its influence on a laboring woman. It is usually more effective to explore the dark corners in the closet than to hope the door stays shut when you least want it to open.

*Courage is the choice to "Do it anyway."*

You may encounter the belief that fear must be resolved before labor can proceed. This is a misconception. Some fears can be dealt with by an explanation from your caregiver and others can't. If fear won't go away, you can choose to allow it to be on the edge of your awareness without letting it direct the show. Fear can be acknowledged without allowing it to immobilize you. Courage is the choice to "Do it anyway."

If you are experiencing fear, in its subtle or more obvious forms, you may be able to access your courage by asking: "What is really happening here? What is needed from me right now?" If you are waiting for the results of a prenatal ultrasound you may be worrying that there might be something wrong with your baby. What is usually true about the present moment is that everything so far has indicated a healthy baby and you need to go on living your life without creating an imaginary problem when you don't know that one exists. If you are struggling through labor contractions you may be concerned that you won't be able to cope if they get any stronger. What is really happening is that you are experiencing a certain level of pain intensity and what you need to do is cope with that level right now. You'll deal with the future when you get there. Worry that expands up to a state of fear is a gradation of intensity that is fueled by fantasizing. Differentiating between what is real and what is imaginary helps you resist the temptation to fantasize, especially when those fantasies are not helpful. It also helps you to avoid escalating up to fear.

During labor women generally are not afraid of the pain that they are currently experiencing, but they do fear that they won't survive if it gets more intense or lasts too long. Maintaining your focus on the present moment and resisting the lure of imagination dramatically improves your ability to cope with intense sensations. It is enough to deal with what is real. Imagination magnifies the perception of the pain's intensity. This is true whenever the body experiences discomfort.

I often suggest awareness of physical sensation as a tool to ground yourself in the present moment. Sensing the weight of your body on your feet or observing your breath gently moving in out and out, helps to bring you back to the here and now. Physical awareness is a lifeline that can pull you back from panic, uncomfortable daydreams, or obsessive thoughts. During labor you may have flashbacks to previous traumatic events. Helping you focus on the sensations in your body or awareness of your current physical surroundings can sometimes bring you back to the safety of the present moment. You also may disassociate from your sense of physical presence when you experience challenging situations. Disassociating in labor rarely acts as an escape from the pain. It is far more likely to disorient you and leave you in a state of chaos. Grounding yourself in the present moment through physical sensations can provide you with the stability to cope with your experience.

✦

I WAS SCARED *by the new and sudden intensity of the contractions in my body, as well as the fact that my midwife wasn't there yet. As a contraction surged and I wanted to leap up and out and away from the pain, my friend calmly reminded me to stay low. I tried to ground the feeling, the pain, myself. "Stay low..." became a repeated mantra as I worked to keep myself from spinning out and checking out. I could do this.*

You can practice working with these two concepts of grounding in sensation and eliminating imagination when you have medical procedures done, such as having your blood drawn. Many women who have a fear of needles report that their usual strategy is to imagine themselves somewhere else and try to ignore what is going on. This decreases your ability to cope with the experience because you are distancing yourself from the reality of the present moment and opening yourself up to imagination. I usually suggest that you try a different approach and actually be interested in feeling the sensation of the needle going into your arm. You can use your emotions in a helpful way by sending nurturing feelings and thanking your body for enduring the discomfort for the sake of the pregnancy and the growing baby. When women use this approach they usually report an overall better experience and less pain. The pain you are imagining is far greater than the reality of what the nerve endings are communicating to the brain. This is an important lesson to take into labor when the pain can be so intense. Falsely magnifying it may have a profoundly negative effect on your ability to cope with it.

*Falsely magnifying pain may have a profoundly negative effect on your ability to cope with it.*

## When Fears Become Reality

While truly dangerous situations or undesirable outcomes don't often arise during childbirth, it is still useful to be able to cope no matter what happens. If you can't change what life brings you, your best choice is to survive it as well as you can. This is when your courage is needed, not to calm down an imaginary fear, but to actually face what you didn't want to encounter. In situations where women are being rushed into an emergency cesarean birth because the baby's heart tones are indicating it is in trouble or families are standing around their newborn's bed in

*If you can't change what life brings you, your best choice is to survive it as well as you can.*

an intensive care unit, I have seen inner strengths emerge in people that they didn't know they possessed. This is when you need to find your stability, clarity, and guidance in your physical, mental, and spiritual centers. Your emotions need to be acknowledged and experienced but they are often not the best leaders in a crisis. Courage gives you the strength to direct your attention to what is needed and provides you with the effort to persevere.

## When Fears Arise from the Past

For some women the fears and anxieties that arise in pregnancy are related to previous traumatic events in their lives. Physical, emotional or sexual abuse, or trauma can have effects later in life on a woman's emotional and physical experiences of pregnancy, birthing, and parenting. (Tallman, Herring 1998) Associations from these experiences may contribute to a vague sense of unease that can be difficult to clarify and resolve. They may be triggered by some aspect of maternity care or experience and be unrelated directly to what is actually going on. Possible examples of these triggers include the relative unpredictability of birthing, the experience of pain, the vulnerability that comes as part of labor, issues around safety, and being physically touched or the necessity of asking for or receiving support.

*Sometimes, having encountered shadows in life can teach you survival skills that you forget to appreciate.*

It has been suggested that perhaps it is better for survivors of abuse and trauma to avoid stirring up old emotional issues with the challenges of birthing and, instead, just schedule cesarean section deliveries. Studies don't support this viewpoint. Instead, they show that women who work to get in touch with their fears coming from past traumas have a more positive experience in their birth regardless of the type of birth they have, vaginal or cesarean. Sometimes, having encountered shadows in life can teach you survival skills that you forget to appreciate. You may

66

not even recognize those skills until you're pressed up against a wall and need them.

✦

*Pregnancy, birth, and breastfeeding have all been opportunities for me to heal and grow. Part of my identity as a healthy sexual being was stolen from me as a young child by the sexual abuse I experienced. Feeling the power of pregnancy shook my core. Giving birth empowered me. Breastfeeding strengthened me. No one was going to take away these opportunities to experience the awe of what my body could do. No one was going to enforce their will on me or my baby. The trust I felt for the midwives offered the safe space for me to birth my daughter and birth my new identity as a mother full of sexuality and healing energy.*

*I learned the more women think that birth is to be feared, then the more the birth experience will be one of trauma and out of their terms. The more women think of the birth experience as a healthy right, then the more the experience will empower women to take birth back into their own homes and hearts. This is so important for us as mothers because it is the beginning of the relationship to our new child and our new lives as teachers.*

Another group of women report worries that arise from knowing too much about the possible undesired maternity outcomes. There are two main subgroups. One is maternity care providers such as labor and delivery nurses, midwives, or obstetricians who have been exposed to the wide range of birth outcomes in their occupations. The other is women who have had previous experiences such as miscarriages, difficult births, breastfeeding challenges, or postpartum depression. They have walked through the door of the unlikely outcome and for them it was their reality; not just a potential. For all of these women, their challenge is to stay grounded in the reality of the healthy pregnancy that they are currently experiencing. The fact that they are more familiar with a potential risk does not necessarily mean it is more likely to happen. They have traded some of the ignorance with which most first time mothers move through pregnancy; but they can be stronger in the understanding that they can deal with complications and can survive them.

APPROACHING MY LABOR, *I became increasingly focused on the "what-ifs." As a midwife and former labor and delivery nurse, I had professional experiences that had exposed me to not only the triumphs of birth and all that happens seamlessly and without intervention, but, also, to the rare experiences where intervention is necessary and lifesaving for mom or baby. My inner work was learning to believe that birth could "work" for me; finding a way to believe that rare things happen rarely; that I wouldn't be the one-in-one-million person who had something devastating happen to me or my baby. I had hoped for an unmedicated birth, but more than anything I was intensely focused on a safe birth, where I felt listened to; and that intervention would not be applied without absolute reason. The "Inner Work of Birth" helped me realize what was truly important to me in my birth: to vocalize what my true apprehensions were to my spouse and myself, and to approach birth as an event that would be my own experience. No matter what that was, it would be valid, unique, and perform its intended purpose: making me a mother.*

I have found that assisting women prenatally in their ability to emotionally cope with their fears regarding birthing and parenting gives them the tools to help heal over-reactive responses and the effects of past traumas. When you call on your courage to face your fears and differentiate reality from imagination you grow in self-confidence and come into contact with your own capabilities as a mature woman. It is not always easy to face your past, but the transformation into motherhood offers you an opportunity to move forward into personal growth and healing.

Libby came to us as a twenty-three year-old in her first pregnancy. She told us she was an extremely anxious person and spent much of her pregnancy concerned with what might go wrong. Her husband was her only family member who believed that she was capable of enduring the pain of labor. She was repeatedly told that she might as well plan on an epidural since she was a "wimp about pain." Throughout our many discussions on the topic, she asserted that she wanted to experience birthing her own baby as fully as possible and she wanted to avoid the use of unnecessary interventions, including pain medications. Multiple discomforts throughout her pregnancy provided many chances to practice working with pain. She reacted with a high level of distress, both in coping with the physical discomforts and in worrying that they might indicate something serious was wrong. When I labor did begin, I was surprised at how well she was coping with the contractions. I checked her cervix and it was four cm dilated. Labor progressed with a gradual increase in the intensity of the contractions. When she got to seven cm dilation, her determination faltered and she became desperate. She kept crying, "I can't do this. It hurts too much. I'll never make it." I asked her to look me in the eyes with each contraction and what I saw there was pure terror. She hung onto my gaze like a tenuous lifeline, struggling to keep from falling back into panic. I couldn't see the dragons that were so frightening to her; but I could feel what effect they had on her. I met her terror with calm confidence and murmured soft words about staying with it and taking one moment at a time. For two hours our gazes were locked with every wave of intensity that swept through her. Her eyes never softened, nor did her attention waver from the support I was sending her. Finally, she was completely dilated and began pushing.

This was an activity that she found much easier than passively accepting the earlier contractions. Thirty-five minutes later she birthed her daughter. She beamed with self-satisfaction and said, "I can't wait to tell my mother I did it!" Later, I reflected on what I had witnessed during her labor. I don't

*Courage often doesn't come when we look our best, but, rather, when we need it the most.*

believe I've ever been as scared as she was and I wonder if I would have had the courage to keep going like she did. Tears came to my eyes as I honored the magnitude of the effort that she had made to hold onto her courageous determination. Courage often doesn't come when we look our best, but, rather, when we need it the most.

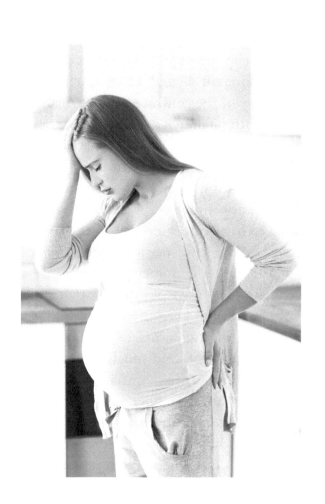

力

# Willingness

*Intense pain will put you face to face with a sensation in your body that, in the moment, most of us would not choose to be experiencing. In that moment something has to be bigger, more important, than the pain. What is it that motivates you enough to not have your way about what the pain feels like?*

## Where Do You Have Choice and Possible Influence in Labor?

There are four main factors that combine to determine the ease and efficiency of how labor progresses. The first is how strong the uterine contractions need to be to push the baby downwards, opening the cervix and causing the head to descend into the vagina. Contractions early in labor tend to be much milder than those later when the cervix is opening to its largest diameter. This is the normal process of labor. You can think of it as climbing a staircase where each step has a greater change in height than the last one. The strength of the contractions a woman experiences when her cervix is halfway open at five centimeters is not strong enough to dilate her cervix fully open to ten centimeters. It is tempting when you are feeling the five-centimeter contractions to tell yourself that you will just continue at the current level of intensity and eventually you will be fully dilated. It doesn't happen like that. If the contractions don't increase in intensity for the next twelve hours you will probably still be at five centimeters when there is another vaginal exam. If your body doesn't increase the strength of the contractions on its own, there are some interventions that may help. These may include changing your position, walking, herbs, homeopathy, acupuncture, breast stimulation (pumping the breasts may stimulate your body to release Oxytocin which increases contractions), or an IV medication called Pitocin that is the synthetic version of Oxytocin. Not all of these methods are available in either an out-of-hospital setting or in-hospital.

The second factor that effects labor progress is the size and position of the baby. The size of the baby is often not something you have a say about; especially once labor starts. Significantly bigger babies usually take more time and work to deliver than smaller babies, unless you have already birthed a few babies previously. Earlier in the pregnancy it is helpful to eat well in order to maintain an appropriate weight gain and a normal blood sugar level. Simply put, this means limiting sweets and junk foods and balancing proteins, fats, and carbohydrates. Otherwise, your baby's genes and the length of time he/she stays growing inside your uterus determine his/her size. The position of the baby once labor starts is something that we may or may not influence. The optimal position that presents the smallest part of your baby's head to fit through the birth canal is with the chin tucked to the chest, facing your back and the head not tilted sideways towards one shoulder. Babies often change position on their own during labor to find the best fit. If they don't get to the best position, it doesn't always mean that they can't be born vaginally but it may take more work. We can sometimes influence babies to rotate to a better position by asking the mom to move to different positions, or by a provider rotating the baby's head with fingers or a hand from inside the vagina. In either of these options the baby has to cooperate in order to be successful.

The third factor influencing the flow of labor is the physical design of the mother's pelvis and birth canal. There is a wide range in the sizes, shapes, and flexibility of these parts in different women. This includes bones, muscles, and soft tissue. The joints of the pelvis stretch to allow more room between the bones while the muscles and soft tissue release to the pressure from the contractions. While pregnancy changes these parts significantly to allow them all to expand, women's bodies do this to different degrees. The first time a woman births vaginally it usually takes more effort on her part to push her baby out. Bodies have a wisdom of their own. Once they have birthed a few babies they usually seem to figure out how to make the process more efficient and quicker. If a baby is having a tight fit, causing labor to not progress, there isn't a lot we can do to change the passageway that the baby has to travel. Allowing more time for the pelvis to expand or changing a mother's position to create different angles inside may do the trick. Sometimes adding an epidural to block the pain sensations may allow the muscles to relax, making more room.

The last factor that can effect a labor's progress is the inner emotional and psychological state of the laboring woman. This is where you have the biggest chance of influencing the course of labor. When you maintain a positive response towards your experience, no matter what it is, you optimize the chances for smooth sailing or for weathering out the storm if that is what shows up. What this may look like is welcoming the contractions as they grow stronger instead of resisting them, accepting the sensation of the pain instead of objecting to it, or adapting to the need for interventions if they become necessary. You need to step up to the plate, take on the responsibility of hitting the ball, and swing with the full intention of bringing in a home run. When this is who you are when you show up for labor, it may improve your chances of compensating for obstacles that may arise from the other factors influencing the birth journey. It is also critical to understand that some labors need interventions no matter how much positive energy a woman pours into her efforts. Sometimes uteruses just

*When you maintain a positive response towards your experience, no matter what it is, you optimize the chances for smooth sailing or for weathering out the storm if that is what shows up.*

need the help of Pitocin. Sometimes babies won't turn to a position that will fit through their mother's vagina. These are times to remember that it is just as important to be flexible as it is to be strong. When you release your original picture of what you wanted in your birth experience and embrace what is needed, you continue to contribute a positive influence on the birth process.

## Making choices and decisions

Most parents care a lot about the many choices and decisions that are part of their pregnancy and birth experiences. Some want a great degree of input and others prefer to follow their provider's suggestions without much questioning. Everyone shares the sense of deep importance that they make the best decisions they can. Seeing the reality of a situation from a broad perspective helps to weigh the options until you find the choices that are right for you. Choosing towards something rather than looking for a way out or avoiding dealing with the situation, keeps you as an active participant in the creation of your child's birth—and, by extension, your life.

✦

> I WANTED TO AVOID STRESS; *I wanted a calm environment. It may sound horrible, but for me this meant not having my mother-in-law attend the birth. She doesn't like me very much and has given me negative comments about how I parent. I knew having her at the birth would make me very uneasy and stressed.*

A significant part of making the best choice is differentiating between what can be changed and what can't. It's wisdom that allows you to do that well. When people don't have a lot of experience in a situation, they often consult experts who know more than they do for advice. What a professional can usually offer you is information. This often helps to get a clearer picture of what is possible and what isn't. However, remember that wisdom is more than just information or knowledge. It also includes intuition, your sense of integrity, and knowing where your true path lies. This becomes especially relevant when you face the challenges of birthing. Only you can choose how you respond to the experience you are having in labor. For laboring women who have difficulty making decisions, this is one you can't get out of. When the contractions become overwhelmingly powerful, you have three possible responses: You can choose to work with the experience (cope with the pain), resist the experience (fight the pain), or change the experience (have an epidural or IV narcotics).

## Expectations and the Unexpected

If you look carefully, you may realize that most moments of your life are shadowed by the expectation of what you believe will happen. When you go to bed at night you expect that you will wake up in the morning. When you are driving to work you expect that the drivers around you will all stop when the light turns red. When you get pregnant you expect that you will end up raising a child. Expectations are the glue that holds the patterns of your life together. They help to hold the chaos at bay. Most of us use them to attempt to steer our life experiences in the directions we want. In something as significant as the birth of a baby, it would be the rare individual who truly could be free of expectations about the event.

*If you are someone who likes to be in control, pregnancy, labor, and parenting may offer you many opportunities to stretch yourself to try flexibility and adaptability instead.*

If you are someone who likes to be in control, (join the club, there are lots of us out here!), pregnancy, labor, and parenting may offer you many opportunities to stretch yourself to try flexibility and adaptability instead. Babies and young children have more freedom from expectations than we do, maybe because they do more things for the first time. While plans and predictability certainly have their value in the maternal and parental world, they can turn into rigidity without some softening and willingness to adapt. Visualizations and goals are valuable, but if they get in the way of what is really needed for the wellbeing of all, they block you from getting where you need to go. A suggestion to work with letting go of control might be to write your birth *preferences*, instead of a birth *plan*.

✦

I TRIED NOT TO MAKE TOO MANY PLANS *for how things would happen once the baby was born. We knew we wanted to co-sleep, and then would be open to adjust, depending on how things were going. I also had picked out some great BPA-free glass bottles and a breast pump so our baby could have breast milk when I was away. Well, what little plans I made went right out the window. We have a wonderful, amazing baby who won't sleep on any flat surface and who absolutely refuses to take a bottle! So, we've adjusted life accordingly – we bought her a curved hammock bed and I changed my schedule around so I'm rarely away from her. It's been a little difficult with her not taking a bottle. I'm hoping she'll be ready for some food and a sippy cup by six months, but I've learned I can't plan for that either!*

You are often not aware of the expectations you carry until an unexpected event makes you confront them. Take a moment to reflect on how you might deal with any of the following unexpected circumstances in labor:

❖ Labor not starting on its own, resulting in the recommendation for induction of labor.

❖ Medical interventions becoming necessary, such as the need to increase your contractions with Pitocin or transport from a home birth.

❖ Complications of labor that require a change of plans towards a cesarean delivery.

❖ Baby not being completely stable when born and needing to spend time in the neonatal intensive care unit.

- ❖ Not getting the support you thought you would have in labor.

- ❖ Not liking being in the water, despite your plans for a water birth.

- ❖ Labor lasting longer than you thought it would.

This list is not intended to frighten you or undermine your self-confidence. Remember, most labors progress normally. We all hope for smooth journeys into parenthood. But thinking that, somehow, you can force your way through to normalcy contradicts the submission that the birthing energy asks of us. Reading the above list and responding with the willingness to take on whatever is needed to birth your baby, affirms a much greater strength than a more superficial need to stay in control.

> *Thinking that, somehow, you can force your way through to normalcy contradicts the submission that the birthing energy asks of us.*

✦

SHORTLY BEFORE MY DUE DATE *I went for my first ultrasound. The doctor who did the ultrasound said, "Your midwife's not going to like this." I was panicked but he wouldn't say more. When I finally saw my midwife she told me I had a placenta previa. This meant that the placenta had implanted over the opening of the uterus and there was no way the baby could safely be delivered vaginally. I would have to have a cesarean delivery. I was numb at first. I cried. I felt cheated out of an experience I had begun thinking of as a challenge I would meet. I knew I could handle the birth as I had handled any other athletic endeavor. I now had to handle the disappointment of having a surgical birth. It was exactly what I didn't want. I tried to meditate on acceptance, letting go of expectations, all the rest. I was more worried about a surgery than I had been about the birth. It felt like I was being forced to let go of control. I had to accept that this was my child's process, not mine.*

# Requiring More of Yourself

One of the most important inner qualities to cultivate in the pathway towards natural birth, is the ability to willingly do what you don't want to do when you have no other choice. This often requires that you to maintain a wider perspective than your immediate desires. For example, most of us would not choose to experience intense pain repeatedly over a span of hours if there were no purpose in it. It is easy to lose your connection to why you are choosing to experience the full reality of labor pain. In that moment, something has to be bigger, more important, than the pain. Something has to motivate you that is of such high value that you are willing to let go all control of what the contraction feels like in your body. When this motivation is directed towards the higher qualities of who you are as a human being, you are capable of performing miracles. Surely, the birth of a new human into life vibrates with

> *Strength of willingness is demonstrated when you realize that some things are greater than you are, and it is an honor to play your small part.*

an energy that is not easily confused with the mundane affairs of the world. You have a place inside yourself that recognizes this. From there you can understand that the work of labor requires far more of you than you would usually ask of yourself.

## Strength of Willingness and Strength of Will

In our society the concept of "strength of willingness" is less familiar than "strength of will." Willingness is essential to the healthy maintenance of any relationship. It comes from the part of you that stops to ask, "How is my action being received?" and "What is needed from me now?" Willingness allows you to adapt and persevere. It often takes a longer, slower road than will but some journeys never reach their end without it. People sometimes confuse the ability to bend, to become what a situation requires, as "giving in." When you live your life always in control and having to have your own way, the capacity to change course mid-stream or follow someone else's advice might be perceived as a weakness. However, stepping back into a bigger picture, the work of willingness can be recognized as a powerful force in the world. It shares a similar energy to water flowing around a boulder in a stream; to the patience of a cocoon waiting to become a butterfly. Its strength is demonstrated when you realize that some things are greater than you are, and it is an honor to play your small part. It is strength of willingness to step forward into the work of birthing a baby without knowing exactly what that might entail.

✦

THE ENERGY OF GIVING BIRTH *is like being on a one-way street. Rivers flow in one direction. Surrendering to this life force energy is what allowed me to have an intense, beautiful, and empowering birth. In this way, there was no room for fear, panic, or any feeling of "I can't do this"...why swim upstream?" With loving support from my partner, sister, and the midwife team, I was able to welcome my son into the world exactly the way I hoped to.*

The first stage of labor, when the contractions grow increasingly stronger to expand the opening of the uterus, is usually the time when willingness is most required. It is a time of patience, perseverance, releasing, and allowing. The neck of the uterus, called the cervix, usually starts labor tight and closed. With time, it submits to the force of the contractions, becoming soft and open. This is a release from deep inside you. You can't command it, control it, or force it. You must be willing to give the birth energy space inside your body to let this process happen; to allow yourself to be inhabited in such a way.

✦

WHEN LABOR CAME, *I really didn't know what to expect. As contractions came and intensified, I turned to yogic pranayama breathing. But this took me away from the contraction and separate from the experience. With guidance, I started relating to each contraction, viewing it as a normal sensation rather than something "to get through." I worked with the wave of energy as it came, feeling that energy move through me like surfing on an ocean wave. I began to cope with the contractions more easily.*

*With time came the need to push. It was the most intense physical sensation I've ever experienced. I went deep inside myself, inside the intensity and used the energy that was there to birth my son. From the depths of myself and through the intense sensation inside, I also gave birth to a more powerful me.*

This is not to say that strength of will is wrong or has no place in labor. In fact, most labors could not be completed without strength of will. Will is more associated with an individual taking ownership and manifesting his or her personal force into the world. There is a dramatic, driving quality to will. It is a force with which to be reckoned; that gets things done. Will isn't about gathering energy; it's about spending it. It shares a similar energy with a lion charging its prey, a crocus pushing up through the spring soil. Strength of will is not always about having your own way. When you find the willingness to change course in labor and do what needs to be done, it may take the focused effort of will to manifest the "doing" part.

✦

WHEN I WAS PUSHING *I felt like I would split in two. But to truly get the necessary force, I had to wait for the contraction, feel the overwhelming compulsion to push, take a breath in, hold my breath, and push even though I was sure I was going to break myself. I kept running out of juice before the third push and would feel the head go back in. Each time I hoped it would come out, whatever it was. I was in primal tunnel vision mode and I don't think I even knew it was my baby anymore. I felt the stinging three times before the head came out. I was so overwhelmed I couldn't look for a second. I said get it out, get it out, as I felt my midwife smoothly slip out the shoulders. Then I saw my baby and I straight up could not believe it. My mind melted off, right then and there.*

The second stage of labor happens once the cervix has been opened and the baby's head is starting to come down into the vagina. It is shorter than first stage and ends with the birth of the baby. This is when strength of will needs to come forth and sound its arrival. Pushing a baby out, particularly for the first time, usually requires an effort beyond what most women have ever done. It requires focus, determination, commitment, and acceptance of the responsibility that this is your job. There's nothing small about it. While your uterus does about half the work, the rest is up to you. You will find strength you never knew you had. This is where you must actively participate or the job doesn't

*Pushing a baby out requires focus, determination, commitment, and acceptance of the responsibility that this is your job. There's nothing small about it.*

get done. Some women are relieved to be done with the allowing energy of first stage and finally get to swing into more focused action. Others may feel a bit reluctant to take on what appears to be so monumental a task. In the end, most women find what they need from inside themselves to push their baby out into the world.

✦

I WAS FOCUSING SO MUCH ON LETTING GO, *jumping off the cliff, that I was surprised when they told me to push hard. I had a hard time figuring out how not to just let go. You have to have both kinds of energy.*

The combination of the right uses of willingness and will create a perfect balance throughout the birth process. Willingness in the first stage of labor is part of what allows you to sustain your effort through the long hours it takes to allow your cervix to open. It is useful to pace yourself and not get too worked up in the beginning part of labor. This can be challenging when you feel the excitement that the day has finally arrived and the race has begun. Be careful about jumping out of the starting gate at full speed. Many women are surprised that while the waiting for labor to begin is finally over, they often find themselves face-to-face with now waiting for the labor to be over. Willingness is needed to allow the process to take the time it takes. Stay in the moment. Do what is in front of you.

The duration of second stage is usually much shorter than first stage. The effort needed during pushing is not the time for energy conservation. This doesn't mean that you necessarily will be pushing to the max with every contraction. Listen to your body and respond honestly. If you're making progress and the baby is descending down your birth canal, keep doing what you're doing. If your baby is not moving, you might want to pause for a check to see if some part of you is holding back. If so, turn up the throttle, full steam ahead. It is important to rest completely between contractions and gather your strength for the next effort. When it comes, meet it with everything you've got. You have what it takes. Believe in yourself. Know that crossing that finish line will be one of the greatest moments of your life. Every push brings your baby closer to your arms. Make every one count. You will find a strength is available to you that you may never have known existed. Keep your bottom loose and be part of the power that brings your baby down and out into the world.

*Meet it with everything you've got. You have what it takes. Believe in yourself. Know that crossing that finish line will be one of the greatest moments of your life.*

✦

I STRUGGLED WITH MY LABOR. *I was sleep deprived, making me irritable and antsy. I am not a passive person, and I had a hard time accepting the pain. I wanted to move forward and feel real progress. When it came time to push I felt so relieved. I became an active participant. I got to do something. I remember looking in the mirror and seeing my baby's head get closer and closer. My excitement was indescribable. Whether I laughed aloud or not, I do not know, but I do know my whole body laughed on the inside as he slipped out.*

# Letting Go of Control

Once you accept that birth is bigger than you are, you can stop fighting it. When pain becomes your ally instead of your enemy, possibilities open up to you that were closed before. For those of us who like being in control this is a change of perspective that may take some convincing. That's okay. Birth has been doing this for a long time. She can wait until you're ready to choose your real role in the process. From a human perspective it is a glorious, incredible role; but to Birth we are the vessel and she is the captain. She determines the course and we do the sailing.

✦

> ALTHOUGH I SPENT A LARGE PORTION OF MY PREGNANCY *terrified about how this little being would make his entrance in the world, many things helped. One, was our support group/class where we could openly talk about our feelings. Two, was time. I had pretty rotten nausea for the first three months and despite every effort I made to make that feeling stop (daily acupuncture, vitamin B shots, constant cracker eating), nothing helped but time. I think that was a good lesson for me; that I could not avoid being in my body even if the experience was painful, and the best I could do was go with it.*

Women often tell me that the reason they are choosing to birth naturally is that they don't want to lose control of the process. The truth is that the real control lies inside you rather than the external events that everyone else sees as labor. It is a control that is reached by being willing to experience the reality of the moment without judgment or having your own way about how it turns out. This requires a paradox of active surrender and passive control. As the contraction pain intensifies or if unexpected events arise, it takes greater and greater effort to surrender into the powerful state of passivity. All of the work that you pour into staying in control is now channeled into letting go and choosing to be where you are. Tremendous change can happen when you keep in touch with one quiet spot inside. Then you can let go and never lose yourself. Freedom from pain is found in the willingness to experience the sensation of the pain in whatever form it takes; in how intense it feels, how long it lasts, how frequently it happens. By trying to limit pain, escape it, or actively control it in any way the muscles tense, making the contractions *more* painful and lengthening the time it takes to do the work.

✦

> THE BIRTH PROCESS REINFORCED MY BELIEF *that I can be strong through ceding control. Earlier in life, I had a very simplistic view of control as an active force that I must manage. As I have grown older— and one hopes, wiser—I have learned that in many circumstances, the best way to maintain "control" is simply to let go. Birth represented an ultimate test of this theory.*

## Floating in the Birth Zone

"Floating in the Birth Zone" is a technique that I have developed through years of working with laboring women to guide them past the point where the pain feels overwhelming and they are ready to give up. Its purpose is to guide them to the choice of existing during a contraction in a state that is boundless.

When most women experience intense pain they eventually come up against a belief that they have encountered the edge of their capacity to cope. I call this the "wall of pain." Women instinctively pull back from it when the contraction hits the peak of its intensity in an effort to protect themselves. The belief tells them that beyond the wall terrible things could happen. They could lose consciousness or break apart. It doesn't matter that it isn't logical. It comes from a feeling of unknown danger. When I describe the wall, women understand what I am talking about. I explain that, in reality, the wall is an illusion based on a false belief. I ask them if they are willing with the next contraction, instead of pulling back from the edge of the pain, to lean into the wall and release themselves through to the other side. For those who accept my proposal, the illusion of the rigid wall dissolves and they find themselves in a state of boundlessness. This dissolving is the result of new beliefs emerging about what they are capable of and who they are.

I then ask women to experience themselves in a state of liquification, where all sensations are acceptable. It is as though they let themselves come apart and stop trying to hold themselves together. Concepts that often are effective in staying in this state are to agree with the sensation, absorb the pain, accept the experience. Instead of struggling with what the contraction wave does to them, I suggest they be the wave. Women usually become quieter and more inwardly turned. They report that it's not that the pain hurts less; it's more that they've stopped fighting it and have found their way back to coping with it. This state of boundlessness allows for change on many levels—from a fetus into a baby, from a woman into a mother. Without the solidity of form pressing in so close around them something happens that is an essential piece to true transformation. After the birthing journey is completed there is a re-solidification into more mature women. Birthing from the highest place in themselves provides them with the opportunity to be closer to who they want to be.

> *Agree with the sensation, absorb the pain, accept the experience.*

✦

I HAD BEEN LABORING FOR HOURS *when my midwife checked me. Six centimeters, 90 percent, baby's head at zero. Then I really disappeared. I had no doubts or questions and I didn't speak to anyone—I only moaned and opened. My partner asked later if I found a position that made me more comfortable, because I stopped moving around or asking him to press on my back or hold me. I said, "No, I just stopped trying to get comfortable, stopped trying to change it, and let the contractions be the reality." At one point, deep into labor, I remember saying, "There is so much pressure down there!" Mostly just to get it out in the open, I think. When I think now about the noises I was making, it seems like they were the sounds—the vibrations—of the contractions themselves. Like, if I had to hold them in, the contractions would be stuck and couldn't do what they needed to do.*

Three guidelines are useful when "Floating in the Birth Zone".

- ❖ First, ground yourself in the present moment with sensation. This opens the doorway through imagination that comes from fears.

- ❖ Second, observe the pain without judging it. This opens the doorway through resistance that comes from judgments.

- ❖ Lastly, surrender your control of the process. This opens the doorway through expectations that come from the need to control.

## Birthing Visualization

As the contraction starts I let my courage sweep me past my limits and into the wave of sensations. I float in the freedom of this experience as long as the contraction is with me. I stay in the present moment and witness the sensations in my body. I know that there is no limit to what I am capable of experiencing. This state is boundless. Some part of me observes and honors the power of the birthing energy which fills my body and I merge to become one with it. I willingly open every door in my body where this energy desires entrance. I allow it to change any part of me that it seeks. The birthing energy is wise in the ways of transformation. I trust that I am protected in this place, as laboring women have been throughout the centuries.

力

# Acceptance

*Coping is in the middle of the pain, the fatigue, the disappointment—they are included. It is not an escape. It is experiencing the disturbance from a higher level inside yourself. Coping doesn't negate the disturbance—it changes your experience of it.*

The third step towards a fulfilling birth experience involves the issues of acceptance and resistance. This duality can be found in the contrast between the following phrases: "I want this; I don't want that" verses "I accept what comes." Acceptance is the space where reality is fully experienced and trusted for its perfection. When you resist something your first step is to judge what is desirable and what is undesirable. When you are motivated through resistance or avoidance you spend your energy either fighting or running away from what you judge to be unpleasant. Instead, fostering a motivation for birth that values acceptance opens doorways that are closed as long as you are stuck in judgment. You are only really free to actively participate when you acknowledge the elements that you can't control and accept what is. Then choices arise within your inner experience that weren't possible before.

It doesn't matter how one asks for *or doesn't ask for help, what stories we have to tell or even how we feel after an event, but what matters is that we show up wholeheartedly. Things get scary and as a mother I know I will continue to be pushed to trust the process and accept the indefinite of this life. And, can I accept myself, even when I'm not proud of who or how I am being? Can I accept the bumps, the bruises, the moments of frozen terror? Can I accept the uglies, the stories I'm ashamed to share? And can I accept my sons as they move forward, sometimes proudly, sometimes in fear, sometimes with help and sometimes on their own? I want to shout a resounding "yes" and I am ready to give myself a break. I am living life the best I know how. I birthed my boys and now I'm parenting them with love, questions, stumbles, and very proud moments. It's an awesome journey and there's no right or wrong... whether I'm depressed or peaceful as a new mama. It's all a process and I'm on board. 110%.*

# Judgments

Judgments are often not easy to discuss. They are hard to talk about without sounding "judgmental!" It may be helpful to remember that they are the basis of any resistance we manifest. Of course, there are times when we need to fight back and strive to change the course of our lives. However, birthing and parenting are full of situations where we simply don't have a choice and resistance is a waste of energy. Swimming upstream is rarely called for in labor.

I was talking to the baby *as I felt my vulva tear – "momma's definitely gonna need stitches, baby." I remember laughing at one point – then laughing about laughing because I never would have guessed that would be possible – to laugh, while giving birth.*

People are often surprised to hear that judgments can be stumbling blocks in birthing. Part of this might be due to the tendency to justify our judgments as, simply, "the right way to think." It takes intentional effort to question our attitudes and opinions in order to begin exploring beyond what we have already decided is true. Judgments can effectively act as buffers with which we hide the truth from ourselves. No one wants to see themselves as judgmental and, yet, if we look closely, we are all in a continual process of assessing what should or shouldn't be happening through most of our lives.

The following is a list of examples that may aid in recognizing how judgments may creep into your experiences of pregnancy, birthing, and parenting:

❖ "Why are my thighs getting so much fatter when the baby is only growing in my belly?"

❖ "How much longer do I have to wait until this baby decides to come?"

❖ "Labor contractions shouldn't hurt this much."

❖ "I ended up having a 'failed home birth' when I had to transport to the hospital during labor."

❖ "I have to breastfeed my baby. What would everyone think if I gave her formula?"

❖ "Every time I set my baby down he cries. What's wrong with him?"

## Polarity and Oneness

An important part of understanding judgments is to recognize that they only exist in polarity. It's like a stick with two ends: Right/Wrong, Good/Bad, Succeed/Fail, etc. The stronger you cling to one side of the polarity and reject the other, the greater you limit the possibilities of what could happen. You can't see the whole picture if you're only willing to examine half of it. When you start to see that the entire continuum has validity you move out of polarity and into oneness. Acceptance exists in the center between success and failure. Another way of expressing this is that acceptance sets you free from defining an experience as either a success or a failure. In embracing both parts of the polarity you transcend the limitations, opening you to higher possibilities. Then you experience a different quality of freedom from which to make your choices.

✦

THE REALITY IS THAT, OVERALL, I FEEL *my son's birth went wonderfully. I didn't even notice that I tore until the midwife told me I was going to need stitches. I said, "Oh, no! I tore? Oh, man... I tore. Stitches? I have to get stitches; It's that bad?" She said, "What are you afraid of?" I paused, "Uh... more pain?" "You just gave birth! This will be nothing." And she was right. It was fine and it didn't hurt being sewn up because she gave me a local anesthetic.*

*The days afterwards were painful at times as I was healing. I was surprised I was so disappointed in my response to tearing. My mind wanted to analyze "what went wrong." Did I push at the wrong time? Did I not do enough perineal massage when I was pregnant? Did I push too hard and too fast? And, I even had thoughts of blame towards my midwife: did she tell me to push harder and more often than necessary? So, I saw my concepts of right and wrong and was pestered with the idea that something must have gone wrong if I tore while giving birth! Eventually, I was able to let this idea go, as I realized it wasn't true.*

One area where judgment often tends to arise is in your choice of focusing on the process or on the results. In order to focus on the process you need to stay in the present moment and do what is needed *now*. The whole maternal experience is seeded with situations in which you are waiting for something to happen: for labor to start, for dilation to be complete so pushing can begin, for the baby to come out, for the baby to stop crying. Impatience arises when you judge that what is currently happening isn't right and something else would be better. The cultivation of patience brings some hope of serenity into the tumultuous journey from pregnancy into parenthood. The results of your efforts will come in their own time. You won't truly know how well you'll do in the parenting process for many decades down the line; and, even then, your influence is only a part of the picture. Life is more about experiencing the journey than about arriving anywhere in particular.

## Anger As Resistance

Another place where resistance can keep you stuck is in various forms of anger. These can range from touchiness, grouchiness, irritability, complaining, yelling; all the ways to tantrums. What they all have in common is that they are fueled by the judgment that something or someone is wrong. This gives you the justification to object and resist. Its voice sounds like, "I won't. You can't make me." There are appropriate places for anger, and this is not a suggestion to suppress it. However, when it blocks progress in labor or when you're trying to soothe a crying baby, anger tends to use up energy that may be better directed towards improving your ability to cope. Women often underestimate the impact that objecting to their experiences in labor has on their perception and coping capacity. Objecting to the pain of contractions creates tension in your body and magnifies your perception of suffering. It may manifest as irritability or, simply, resistance. Questioning the judgment behind the objection can sometimes reveal options of which you were previously unaware.

*The cultivation of patience brings some hope of serenity into the tumultuous journey from pregnancy into parenthood.*

You are only free to choose when you have dissolved the boundaries of judgment and accepted the whole picture of a situation. In order to do this you need to be willing to question your habitual attitudes, opinions, and assumptions that limit your vision. When you accept the whole truth, acknowledging both sides of a polarity, you can come to the center. An example that many women have used in labor can be phrased as, "Isn't easy; isn't hard. Just is."

GETTING PAST THE PAIN, CONFUSION, AND SELF-DOUBT *of breastfeeding was a cycle that took a lot of processing. One powerful message that I received in the "Inner Work of Birth" class was that you can hold the disappointment and hold the joy at the same time. Whenever it felt like a struggle, I remembered that despite the struggle— the joy was real. The discomfort is real, too; but the joy makes it worth it.*

## Your Relationship with Pain

The most common place where resistance arises in labor is in your response to the pain of contractions. One of the most important preparations for a natural birth is to examine your relationship to pain, including your beliefs, attitudes, and expectations. This exploration can include previous experiences with pain, both physical and emotional. Is there a connection between past trauma and the view that the pain of labor must also be traumatic?

DURING MY SECOND PREGNANCY *I realized that my fear of the pain of contractions led to resistance. In my first labor, I was gritting my teeth and just trying to get through it, even though intellectually I knew better than to fight labor. On a primal level, my fear and anxiety led me to resist the power of the contractions, the power of birth. I realized that I was resisting myself and working against the power of my own body to birth my baby. The strong surges of the contractions were created by ME, by MY BODY, to birth MY BABY. I realized that rather than resist, I could go into the power of birth and work with it. Why should I fear the power of my own body?*

*I knew labor would still be intense and strong but that fundamental shift in how I perceived the pain made it more tolerable. In my second labor I used affirmations such as, "Let the power of birth flow through me" to stay in the moment and open to the contractions. I chanted, "Open and down" when they became strong. A little over two hours after my labor started, I birthed my son.*

There is a significant difference between the simplicity of experiencing the sensation of labor contractions (accepting them) and suffering through them (judging them). Suffering adds the judgment that the experience is bad, unnecessary, or shouldn't be happening. When you release the interpretation that the pain is wrong, your ability to cope with it increases dramatically. One of the most effective pain management techniques is the ability to be in the present moment and observe the sensations in your body without judging them. Your choice about pain in a natural labor is in your response to it; not in its intensity or duration. Imagination, coming from fears; and resistance, coming from judgments, magnify the sensation of what is really happening. The simpler you can keep your interpretation of the pain messages that are being sent to your brain; the better you can deal with them. The new mothers at one of our birth class reunions discussed what advice they wished to pass on to other women who were approaching the birth process. Their formulation was: "Take what you get. Do it until it's done."

*Take what you get. Do it until it's done.*

✦

My husband views my role in the births *of our two children similarly: "you were incredible; in control, strong, tireless, magnificent. Don't you feel empowered?" Truth is, after the birth of our first child, I felt traumatized, and empowered was not in my vernacular.*

*We wanted a low-intervention childbirth in order to minimize risk of c-section and to maximize my ability to bond with the baby in the immediate postpartum period. Two factors contributed to the traumatic nature of the birth of our first child: the repeated, unwanted interventions, as well as the way I coped with the less than ideal circumstances of a medicalized birth.*

*At thirty-eight weeks, we were admitted to the hospital after I developed complications from a presumed abdominal abscess related to my Crohn's disease. Several specialists recommended that we have a c-section and exploratory abdominal surgery in the general operating room. We declined both procedures and, instead, elected to be induced. After close monitoring, three days of IV antibiotics for the infection, and multiple induction attempts, labor started and I was already exhausted. The labor was short: five and a half hours in total length.*

The most challenging part of the labor was that I had no break from the contractions, greeting each one with disbelief and, even horror, as they got stronger. Ultimately, I felt disconnected from my body and baby as I grinned and bared each assault. The "don't-push-yet" stage was truly a nightmare. My body told me otherwise, and I suffered greatly trying to listen to instruction. Eventually, my body took over and I could not help but push. Not allowed to deliver in the water, I was transferred from the safety and security of the dimly lit birthing tub room to the bright lights and urgency of the delivery room with a slew of strangers. Forty minutes of hurried pushing and my daughter was pulled from my body, leaving me with horrible pelvic floor tears. Then I had a retained placenta that had to be removed manually (and I had not had an epidural) and needed an hour and a half of stitching. I spent another two and a half hours trying to cope with all that instead of being focused on our new babe.

All in all, I suffered the most, not when I was told I would need a cesarean and an exploratory abdominal surgery; not when we had to repeatedly advocate for ourselves and our baby for a low-intervention birth; not when I was told to push, push, push and my daughter was aggressively pulled from my body; not when my placenta had to be manually removed without an epidural: I suffered the most when I abandoned my body, baby, self, and partner; unsure of how else to cope, as I endured painful contraction after contraction, and was ultimately directed not to push when my body told me otherwise.

After our challenging experience at the hospital, we opted for a homebirth for our second child with local midwives. Our plan was thwarted when our midwife estimated our son to be in the ten-pound range. We revised our birth plan to have our midwives help us deliver in the hospital with a water birth no longer an option. We agreed to be induced in order to maximize our chances of a vaginal delivery in the context of my chronic medical condition. After we arrived at the hospital, a cervical ripening agent was used to attempt to induce labor. Three hours later, I awoke to rip-roaring contractions, contacted our doula, woke my husband, and it was game-on!

In preparation for our second child, I had done substantial work to make sense of the difficult aspects of our daughter's birth. As I labored in the tub for two hours, I centered on the ideas of surrendering willingly to each contraction, visualizing my cervix preparing me for the pushing stage; used cleansing breaths that focused on faith, trust, and gratitude to let go after each contraction and also to center myself as a new contraction approached. My husband and doula helped me to let go of the tension and relax my body between contractions. And suddenly, it was time to push!

I was helped out of the tub and onto all fours to maximize the exit strategy for this large baby of ours. Unlike the birth of my daughter, where the pushing stage felt like a relief and was not the most painful part of the labor; pushing this time was hard! Instead of abandoning my body and baby as I did with the birth of my daughter, I worked hard to stay connected to my body, to ask for reassurance from my birthing team (this is hard for me!), talked to my son, and trusted my body to bring a healthy baby into this world. I used what seemed like every muscle in my body to push for an hour and a half. My husband was everything I needed, as he sat close by and reassured me that I was doing great work. The lovely "ring of fire" lasted entirely too long and just when I began to think it would never happen, after just three and a half hours of rip-roaring labor from start to finish, my husband and I were overwhelmed with emotion and love as we welcomed our son weighing in at a whopping 9lbs 15oz!

The entire experience was everything I hoped for, none of which I was afforded during my first birth experience: including dim lights, a calm, competent, and nurturing birthing team; no sense of urgency; and I felt wrapped in love and adoration throughout the entire process. I took leaps of faith, rendered myself vulnerable, and asked for reassurance when needed. During my first birth, it didn't even occur to me that there was any other way to cope than to go it alone and simply endure each contraction. With my second birth, it was clear to me that I could greet each contraction, welcoming the natural changes in my body that would bring me closer to meeting my son. With the very beginning of each contraction, the cleansing breath I took allowed me to stay connected to my body and baby despite extreme physical discomfort. My willingness to ask for and accept reassurance from my team allowed me to stay connected with them throughout the process as well. In the end, I felt like a COMPLETE ROCK STAR and blessed by my birthing team and husband: the experience was beyond sacred; it was perfect.

# When Epidurals Don't Work

An unexpected situation that women occasionally face in labor is when epidurals don't work. Usually when this happens there is at least partial pain relief and there is only part of the abdomen where the medication fails to block the nerve endings that report pain to the brain. Rarely, women report that the epidural is entirely ineffective at providing pain relief anywhere in their body. Most cases of either partial or complete failures can be remedied and women then experience a level of comfort that is acceptable to them. This is done first by changing the laboring woman's position to encourage the medication to flow where it is needed to get an effect. If that doesn't work, the anesthesiologist is called back and he or she adjusts the levels of medication or the placement of the epidural tube in the woman's back. If these measures aren't effective, the tube is removed and a second epidural is placed to get adequate coverage of the pain sensations. Again, most of the time this will do the trick. The really big challenge comes in those rare occasions when, after hours of trying to get it to work, the anesthesiologist reluctantly says, "That's as good as it's going to get." Usually, by this point, the laboring woman is frustrated, disappointed, and often just plain mad. Nobody on the birth team is happy because the woman is clearly suffering.

This is different from supporting laboring women who are choosing to experience the pain of the contractions. Usually, when a woman has requested an epidural it is because, either she never wanted to experience intense labor pains, or she has already worked with them and has decided that she is done doing it on her own. Most women assume that an epidural will always be an option if they don't want to deal with the pain anymore. There are certainly parts of the world where an epidural is not readily available but the women there don't have the expectation that it would be there if they wanted it. Women who have experienced ineffective epidurals sometimes feel abandoned by the health care system and criticized that they are over-reacting to the pain. A more supportive response by health care providers is to acknowledge to the woman that she experiencing pain that is unacceptable to her and to validate how challenging this situation is. Then, she needs to clearly be told that the epidural coverage just isn't going to get any better. In cases where the epidural is completely ineffective, she has three choices of how to proceed. She can have a cesarean section with a general anesthetic (she would be "put to sleep" with medications throughout the surgery) or she can proceed with a vaginal birth, continuing to suffer, fighting the contractions. Her last option is to also continue birthing vaginally; however, in this case, she would need to accept the sensation of pain and do her best to work with the birth process, releasing her resistance and objections. These three options need to be presented with absolute compassion and free from any judgments. Experiencing pain where we have no choice is how most women through history have gone through labor. The addition of pain medications in the last century requires that women now must make more choices.

✦

MY PLAN FROM THE MOMENT I FOUND OUT *I was pregnant was to have a natural water birth. And, I believed from the very beginning that I was more than capable of enduring the pains of labor. This was just the way it was going to be! I took a hypnobirthing class to learn how to breathe and what it meant to visualize the birth process as it was happening. I read "Childbirth Without Fear" by Grantly Dick-Read, in which he presents his fear-tension-pain theory. I watched countless childbirth videos, most of which were water births. I was dead set on having this baby naturally and no one could change my mind.*

*Time didn't exist while I was laboring. All I knew in those moments was that my contractions were coming every one to two minutes and lasting for what seemed an eternity. Hours went by. Finally, I was checked a second time – I was seven centimeters dilated, eighty-five percent effaced. I wasn't encouraged by this update, but it was progress nonetheless. I entered into the transition stage of labor shortly after this check. From what I was told, there was no progress in cervical dilation in the next six and a half hours—this part of my labor is a complete blur. I was a wreck. I was still at a seven centimeters and the end was nowhere in sight. After a quick ultrasound, we found out that my baby's head was tilted and not engaging with my cervix. This was causing the lull in my progress. After thirty-five hours of labor, I asked for an epidural. The decision was accompanied with a mixture of emotions – disappointment, fear, anxiety, relief, hope. It was not what I had wanted or planned. However, I never imagined my labor would last thirty-five hours. I never considered that my baby might not be positioned correctly.*

*The anesthesiologists came shortly after I made my request. After a brief explanation of the process, the procedure was complete. I started feeling relief in just moments. Then, the relief was only on my left side; there was no change in the right side of my body. The anesthesiologist took out the first epidural and repeated the procedure. Relief. I was able to rest for about two hours. Then my contractions resurfaced and began surging through my body again, one by one. This time, they seemed much more intense. Again, the anesthesiologist came to my room. He tried to increase the dosage of my epidural, but no relief came. He left.*

*I was exhausted, to say the least. There are no words to describe the utter desperation I felt for something – anything. For rest. For the edge to be taken off. For this all to be over. Then my midwife sat at the side of my bed. She looked at me with honesty and explained that there was nothing left for the anesthesiologist to do. He could not offer me any more relief. I had two choices: One, to have a c-section;, but this would need to be an immediate decision and I would need to be taken directly to the operating room, or two; I would need to find a way to calm down, accept the pain, and push this baby out. I took two, maybe three, breaths and chose to push.*

*Thinking back on this decision, I have a hard time pin-pointing the reason I chose to push. I mean, a c-section is clearly the easier choice. My work would be done. I would be wheeled into a sterile operating room, given some kind of anesthesia, and the doctors would hand me my baby a few minutes later. Why would I choose to push?*

*It all comes down to these three things:*

1. *I had made up my mind from the beginning that I CAN do this. I knew I was made to do this. Millions of women had done this before me; and millions more would do this after me. Knowing that I was capable pushed me toward the hard choice. If I was made to do this and I was capable of doing this, then I was going to do this.*

2. *Because I was so set on a natural delivery before ever going into labor, I think I automatically developed a predisposition to believing that a c-section was a bad thing. Reasonably, I understood that c-sections are necessary and good in some situations. But my midwife had given me the option. If I had an option, then it meant that, at this point, a c-section was not necessary. If it wasn't necessary, then I didn't want it.*

3. *My midwife said something so profound in that moment at the side of my bed. She told me to accept the pain. Accept. Not to pretend it wasn't there. But to accept it. Accept the fact that it wasn't going away. Accept the fact that this pain was a part of the process. Accept that this was the only thing holding me back from meeting my baby boy and finally holding him in my arms. It was an easy choice – I accepted it.*

*I pushed. Two hours later an eight-pound, twelve-ounce baby boy was placed on my chest. It was over. The pain was gone. I stepped out of hell and into paradise, and I greeted my son with a clear mind, open arms, and skin-to-skin touch. I would have missed out on all of that if I had made the easier choice. I have not, for even one moment, regretted my decision to push. I felt my baby leave my body – I have nearly forgotten the pain, but I will never forget that.*

In my many years of serving as a midwife, I have come to develop great respect and value for the lessons that pain brings to us. Our hearts and spirits have the potential to grow far more during our times of struggle than our times of peace. We certainly need the nurturing of love and serenity in our lives to give us the sustenance that carries us through our dark nights and rock bottoms. However, when we view pain as our ally, we may find treasures inside ourselves that only pain can reveal. Trusting that life will bring what is needed will help to perceive crises and challenges as interesting lessons and wise teachers. When women bring this truth into their labors; it changes the meaning of their experiences.

> *When we view pain as our ally, we may find treasures inside ourselves that only pain can reveal.*

# What Ifs...

One of the hardest topics to talk about during pregnancy is what happens if one of your "what ifs" comes true? Unexpected or undesirable outcomes are not usual. However, the truth is that they can, and occasionally do, occur. They may include unexpected interventions such as hospital transport from an intended out-of-hospital birth, the use of pitocin, cesarean section delivery, or a baby who ends up needing to be in an intensive care environment. There are babies who are born with congenital abnormalities or experience traumatic events that lead to disabilities; leading people into a different parenting experience from what they had imagined for themselves. Finally, in spite of all of our best intentions, sincere efforts, and modern technology, not all babies who are conceived go on to continue the life cycle that we all expect. Their lives are relatively short—sometimes weeks, ending in miscarriages. Others pass through the birth process only long enough to live for a few hours or days. Their parents are presented with the challenge of accepting the reality that their life together as a family has ended quickly. They must walk the path of both preparing a funeral and storing away the baby clothes that lie waiting at home.

Grieving is a normal and necessary process that follows an unexpected or undesirable outcome. There is a sorrow in the loss of the future that was expected and, somewhere down the road, a struggle to find the value in what came instead. The judgment that something wrong occurred usually arises. Depending partially on how extreme the event was, it may take much time and effort to complete the grieving process and end up in a healthy place of serenity and acceptance. In order to do this, it helps to allow yourself to experience the fullness of your emotions without judgment. If you are having difficulty moving towards a peaceful resolution of grief, it may be appropriate to seek professional guidance.

MY FIRST PREGNANCY AS A SINGLE MOM *and cesarean birth were very difficult for me. During my second pregnancy I was in the "Inner Work Of Birth" class. I had a chance to look at how I carried so many of the pains and worries of bringing my first child into the world and how that seemed to surround my second pregnancy. The class helped me move through those experiences in a more conscious way. I felt insecure telling stories of my first pregnancy, of being alone and afraid, of how I couldn't be pregnant without feeling the weight of my first experience alongside the second. I didn't have the joy and anticipation like the other women, and I wish I could have had that kind of pregnancy experience. Through my pregnancy I had the chance to grieve and heal. I am grateful that I had the chance to do that and at the same time I feel badly that I didn't have the innocent longing for my child that the other moms had. The grieving continued in a profound way for many months and burdened my postpartum depression, sleep-deprived, stressed-out state.*

The temptation to slip into blame is often present when a birth brings unexpected events or outcomes. The difficulty with blaming others is that it disempowers you because you give away responsibility. If you blame yourself you are still trapped in the polarity of right/wrong. Without coming to acceptance you can't perceive your birth experience with self- satisfaction or empowerment. The price of blame is too high to pay for it blocks you from your own inner peace and sense of accomplishment.

The experience of loss related to pregnancy and birth resonates deeply inside you. Most women grow up expecting that if they want to birth babies their bodies will be able to do that. If you find yourself faced with infertility it may feel like a life experience that most everybody else can choose has been stolen from you. It just doesn't seem right that a baby can miscarry before it even has a chance to live on its own or die so soon after birth without ever really seeing what the world is about. While the sadness of these experiences never goes away, there is an unexpected gift that often appears in the parents who have experienced pregnancy or newborn loss. If they are given another chance at pregnancy, there is often an increased gratitude and sense of value if the process works normally—they don't take it for granted in the same way as other couples.

The pathway to peace is acceptance. I will always remember the parents and baby who helped me to clarify this understanding. Their baby entered life with unexpected damage to its brain. She lived for three days. I will be forever touched by the experience of sharing this mother's and father's deep sorrow and my witnessing of their courage in facing what life had brought them. In my efforts to continue to support the parents through the shock and grief of their baby's short life, I realized that the same basic advice we give about coping with physical pain also applies to emotional pain. Allow yourself to feel the sensation or the emotion in a place inside yourself that is free of judgment. Let it be what it is; honoring it as a precious moment in your life that is very real. The fact that you can hurt, both physically and emotionally, is part of the gift of being alive. The wise old women are the ones who didn't turn away when life tore them open. Instead, they stayed there and let themselves be transformed.

> *The wise old women are the ones who didn't turn away when life tore them open. Instead, they stayed there and let themselves be transformed.*

There is no right or wrong way to proceed after losing the life that you thought you would share with your baby. The sadness will probably never go away. Yet with acceptance, it may become a rich and meaningful part of the tapestry of your life. Honoring what is right for you as you move forward into your future reminds you of how precious life is.

◆

I AM THE MOTHER OF THREE CHILDREN, *Rebecca, Eli, and Arielle. Rebecca, my first child, died when she was days old, from what we think was oxygen loss suffered during labor. We have never been able to determine exactly why this happened. I had a normal pregnancy and a normal labor with her. The experience of birthing Rebecca was one of the most profound experiences of my life, and though we had wished to have more children, I know I will never labor in that way again. Rebecca's birth was a home birth. This fact is not related to her demise; however, it is important to mention because it conveys that I had to go through an incredible mental and physical challenge in order to bring her into this world. After she arrived and could not take her first breath, she was rushed to the hospital. She never came home.*

*The first year of mourning Rebecca was unbelievably difficult and very confusing. I became pregnant with Eli three-and-a-half months after Rebecca's death; and this spawned many confusing and sometimes contradictory emotions. I wanted Rebecca, but if I had Rebecca, I wouldn't have the new life inside me; and I wanted this new life inside me, too. I regularly had dreams about vast, desolate places where I wandered feeling vulnerable, and in each of these dreams there was a symbol of hope: I was swimming in an ocean and riding the waves and was nearing the shoreline. I was wandering in an ice-covered region in the nighttime, but there was a beautiful constellation moving across the sky. These were dreams about life prevailing amidst my profound grief.*

*When I became pregnant with Eli, I knew I wanted to have a cesarean section. The process of grieving Rebecca was taking everything I had emotionally, and I couldn't see myself doing the mental work of labor. Also, labor, for me, was associated with what eventually killed Rebecca; and I didn't think I could open myself up to the process. I thought if I did labor, I would unconsciously try to hold this new baby inside me rather than do the mental and physical work to open myself up and dilate. I had lost all control with Rebecca's death and now I needed to know when this child would be born, and how. With Rebecca, I had been almost politically adamant about having a natural birth. Now, I scolded myself for my past self-righteousness: there are many ways to do birth and many reasons women have for choosing to do birth in a different way other than a natural home birth. Before, I had overlooked the work that a woman does over nine months to grow the baby, and had only seen the birth itself as the work needed to bring a baby into the world. This time, I was going to commit myself to those nine months and give myself credit for the immense amount of work needed to do that; and to do it in the midst of profound grief. I would give myself a break on the labor itself.*

*Eli's birth was incredibly special, despite it being under the fluorescent lights of the operating room. My husband sat beside me and we looked into each other's eyes as the doctor opened up my abdomen and pulled Eli out. After I was sown up, the staff wheeled me out to the hallway where our families were waiting, and everyone cried with the relief of seeing our live, healthy baby crying in my arms.*

## Trust

When you are free of the boundaries of judgments you can let go and trust. What is it that needs to be trusted in labor? There are four main areas of focus where the inner state of trusting may open doorways for you in labor. The first is to trust yourself and your own capabilities. We will address this later when we discuss self-confidence in the chapter on empowerment. The second is trust of your support system, your partner, and birth attendants. This will be addressed in the chapter on receiving support. Here we will discuss trust of your body. Finally, in the next section, we will cover trusting the birth process.

✦

THERE WAS A PERIOD *during the middle of my labor when I did not know if I could continue, or how. I felt so exhausted, and also overwhelmed by the unknowing of what was to come. I was still thinking about all that was happening with my conscious mind, and I believe this made it difficult for me to surrender to and trust the natural process I was moving through. After a time of doubting, the physical sensations became so all-encompassing that there was no room left for me to think. After my conscious mind stepped back, I was able to work more productively with the physical process. It was a hot summer afternoon, evening, and night, and I walked for hours back and forth across the wooden floorboards of our porch. What I remember from that time right before my son was born does not involve any conscious thought, but, instead, images and sensations; my solid, bare feet against the floorboards, the late light casting down through a bunch of sunflowers, later the bats darting against the night sky. I felt at one with the wood, the flowers, the sun, the darkness.*

People vary in how much they trust in, or even have a sense of, relationship with their bodies. There are many factors that seem to influence this, including their involvement with physical activities or their personal histories of illnesses or accidents.

Judgment may block a connection with your body by replacing awareness of sensations with evaluating. For example, if a negative judgment from the mind sends the message of a need to protect and defend against the contractions, the body may respond with muscle tension that usually overrides the intent to relax. Instead of working with the birth process, this tension creates resistance that sometimes interferes with labor progress.

An important aspect of trusting your body lies in the area of communication. Your bodily sensations provide important connections to your mind that aid in fully participating in the birth process. Accepting these sensations, without judging them as good or bad, can open up a two-way communication between your mind and body. The body's wisdom can be recognized when the mind listens to the sensations that the body sends. Your body may give you feedback about what's happening in labor to guide and inform you regarding many choices you will make. Examples of this include what positions to labor in or how to push effectively. Sometimes your body can guide you better than your mind can.

The communication can also go in the other direction. When your mind is truly paying attention to your body it allows you to gently make requests than can be beneficial during labor. As a midwife, I utilize this to sometimes get slow labors back on the track of efficiency. For example, a woman's body may respond to subconscious requests to escape pain by keeping the contractions at a low, ineffective level, resulting in hours of regular contractions that aren't changing the cervical dilation. I talk with women about coming back to viewing pain as their ally. When they're ready to pick things up to get some labor work done, I suggest they turn inwards and ask their bodies for increased power and frequency of contractions. When women sincerely do this I often see a dramatic change for the better in the contraction pattern and labor proceeds effectively. I also use the mind-body connection at the first sign of a woman starting to bleed too much after delivery. I tell her to ask her body to tighten her uterine muscles and close off the bleeding blood vessels. As I turn around to give her medications for the hemorrhage, I often find that her body has already responded and slowed the bleeding on its own.

## Trusting the Birthing Process

Another area where trust is useful in labor is in regards to the birthing process. Some women find remembering that women have been birthing babies for millions of years reinforces their belief that "The plan is good." In observing the process for thirty-seven years, I have come to my personal belief that birth has its own wisdom and it works best when we take the time to respect it. As I sit with laboring women, I often sense that there is a sacred universal energy that comes sweeping through their bodies as the contractions rise up within them. Birthing energy has produced an entire planet of people by weaving its way through female bodies. Dance with it. My logical mind can't verify whether this is true or not; but it works for me—and many women can relate to my description of my sense of the sacred. If the concept is too new-age for you, feel free to bypass it. I offer it as another possible way of coping in labor and it may resonate for you.

*Birthing energy has produced an entire planet of people by weaving its way through female bodies. Dance with it.*

One woman's labor stands out as an example of an effective use of this imagery. She was struggling with the pain of the contractions; resisting them, despite her efforts to relax. It had been several hours since her labor had progressed. I suggested she view her body as a vessel that had been given the honor of channeling the sacred energy of birth. This energy had come to bring her child into its own independent life.

Within the span of minutes I watched her change from perceiving the experience as useless suffering into the privilege of participating in a miraculous event. She calmly focused inside herself and her body responded with a smooth progression until her son was handed up into her arms. Other women have turned to their faith in God and trusted that whatever was asked of them in labor was an act of service to the Higher. When we view birthing as part of our spiritual path we bring forth many of our greatest strengths. While the task is rarely easy, when we birth with an awareness of higher meaning we are often capable of much greater efforts.

✦

I FOUND THE EXPERIENCE OF DEEP LABOR *and pushing to be about following the tail of trust down the rabbit hole. The turning point for me came when I stopped trying to get comfortable, trying to find the right position—stopped trying. In a way, I stopped having an opinion at all. I was the way a newborn is: wide open. Or, so I thought. After a few pushes, my midwife said that to get the baby out, I would have to go past what I believed was possible, and I got another lesson in trust. Unlike the rest of the labor, where I worked only to get out of the way, this time I had to trust that I could do it—with my will and strength and determination; but mostly with the willingness that accepted my midwife's advice at the deepest level—chose her view of reality over mine—so that it changed my belief and perception. That was the jumping point, and I landed with a baby in my arms.*

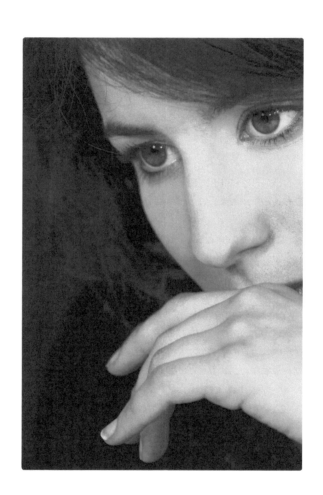

力

# Empowerment

*Pain's intensity can lead you to share in its power
and strength. Who are we to dare to be so powerful?
We are the women who birth the human beings
into life on this planet.*

Pregnancy, birth, and postpartum are times when you are pushed into frequent encounters with vulnerability. Since all of these phases of the maternal experience include processes of transformation, they necessitate the experience of openness and letting go of the familiar. You cannot change a form, including your current state of being and self-identification, without eliminating some of the barriers that provide you with the illusion of security. This leaves you in that soft, unprotected place of vulnerability. If you are strongly invested in controlling your life, this may be one of the greatest challenges of bringing a baby into the world.

## Pregnancy and Vulnerability

You face vulnerability when your privacy boundaries are challenged in regards to your pregnant body. Throughout the pregnancy, your body is frequently exposed and touched by professional caregivers as they palpate the growing baby, draw blood, and do vaginal examinations. About halfway through the pregnancy you become "publically pregnant." Your belly is large enough that strangers can see that you are pregnant and slight acquaintances often take the liberty of touching your pregnant abdomen or commenting on your size. While efforts are made to respect modesty, when it comes to pushing a baby out, it is usually done with your lower body naked and your legs open before a group of people. Your naked breasts will be exposed more during breastfeeding that at any other time of your life.

◆

I EXPERIENCED THE VULNERABLE STATE *that I encountered in labor in a very internal way. The energy inside of me was so big that I had nothing left to devote to what was going on around me. Transition and pushing were such primal, uninhibited places to be in, and it was almost magical the way my fear of being vulnerable and my awareness of being observed just fell away.*

Pregnancy also requires you to experience physical vulnerability. By the third trimester you may find it difficult to bend down to tie your shoes. When you are out alone you may be aware that you couldn't run away to defend yourself if the need arose. If you choose to labor without pain medications you will probably have to walk the path of opening to the intense physical sensations. After the baby arrives, you may face the prospect of having to recondition your body back to your pre-pregnant state of fitness.

Perhaps the area where your soft spot of vulnerability may feel most exposed is in the realm of emotions. Most pregnant women report that their emotions are more sensitive and less easily controlled than when they aren't pregnant. You may not be able to tolerate scary movies or violence on television. In preparing for birthing and parenting, you may find yourself processing sensitive subjects with your caregiver or partner. Labor often brings you face-to-face with emotional issues such as dealing with irrational fears or the conflict between letting go and feeling safe. Once you land into motherhood you discover that not only your daily routine, but, also, your sense of who you are has often changed.

While the examples above may seem a bit daunting, it is important to remember that vulnerability doesn't mean helplessness. Adaptability and the capacity to change are powerful allies in coping with challenges. This is how you can receive and embrace what life brings you. It is possible to grow and become stronger through the opportunities that pregnancy, birth, and parenting provide. This can lead you to the gifts of maturity, serenity, and wisdom. Remember to include softness

*Once you land into motherhood you discover that not only your daily routine, but, also, your sense of who you are has often changed.*

in your picture of strength in labor. Birth is sensuous, slippery, yielding. You are most powerful when you step forward—unprotected and vulnerable. When you have nothing left to lose, anything is possible.

✦

AS A NEW MOTHER, *I've received a heightened sensitivity. My empathy and compassion in nearly all areas feels awakened. Sometimes this feels vulnerable. But through it all, it feels like a gift to see the world with a softer heart.*

## Empowerment

The process of birthing involves moving the physical body of a baby out into the world. Powerful energy is required not only to create the force behind this movement, but, also, to sustain the capacity that completes the process. This involves a different kind of strength than the ability to be vulnerable described above. Parts of labor, particularly the second stage in which a woman pushes her baby out her vagina, require a focused effort. In this, strength manifests as the ability to do, rather than allow. This manifestation of power can be challenging for some women. Others can't wait until they're through the hours of letting the contractions open their cervix and they can get more actively involved in pushing their baby out. The truth is, the effort to allow often takes as much intentional work as it does to actively participate in doing. Women sometimes have a preference as to which seems easier to them.

It is helpful to explore how you relate to expressing power. You may not feel comfortable seeing yourself as powerful if you associate the word with domination. I use the word "power" in a less polarized manner, defining it here as the movement of energy transforming into expression. *Empowerment is the experience of enabling yourself with the energy of power.* There are many ways that you can describe your inner state when you feel empowered. You may talk about strength, determination, perseverance, or courage. This is when you are stepping up and functioning at your full capacity. It leads you to many rich, meaningful experiences in your life. It fills you with the joy of being alive.

> *Empowerment is when you are stepping up and functioning at your full capacity.*

✦

> BEFORE GIVING BIRTH, *I would have pointed to a variety of "achievements" as evoking feelings of empowerment, such as earning an MBA from Harvard, or selling a company, or sailing a boat in difficult conditions. Giving birth trumps them all: It's on a completely different level that makes those "achievements" seem trivial.*

In order to view yourself as a strong, capable human being it is useful to reflect on your own experiences of empowerment. Maturity can bring you the ability to recognize empowerment in situations where, in the past, you failed to give yourself the acknowledgement of what you have accomplished. When I discuss power in birth preparation classes, it sometimes takes a while for women to recognize their own past experiences of empowerment. I ask them, "When have you felt particularly empowered in your life? What were the moments when you felt great about yourself?" The following is a sample of the examples I've heard.

ANY TIME I'M ON STAGE DANCING *I feel empowered. I'm not a very outgoing person and I don't really like being the center of attention in my actual life, but performing allows me to be a different person. I am strong, aggressive, powerful, and casually graceful in my dance.*

Women often give examples of empowerment such as traveling alone or moving a long distance by themselves. They talk about having had to rely on themselves more completely than they had to previously. Sometimes completing a home or car maintenance project is an empowering experience for women who are not the handyman type. Every time they walk by the wall lamp where they drilled the holes to attach the hardware, a little flame of pride lights up inside them. The challenge of athletic events allows many women to experience a sense of power. Recall the sense of presence and determination it takes to step up to the plate and ready the baseball bat as you await the pitch of the ball. Working with animals requires both a respectful and strong inner presence. Women have described sitting on the back of a frightened horse and maintaining their role as the leader. Reaching our career goals rarely happens without perseverance. One woman acknowledged the courage it took to call herself an artist and clear the space in her daily life to manifest her creations. Relationships may present challenges that require women to stand up for themselves. It often takes a great deal of strength for women to leave unhealthy or abusive relationships and face the world alone as a single woman. Our list wouldn't be complete without mentioning the birth stories that always come up when we ask about previous experiences of empowerment. Our repeat moms often describe their labors as one of the most intense experiences with power in their lives—both in their inner state and in being connected with something bigger than themselves.

*I'VE BEEN A PROFESSIONAL MUSICIAN for 15 years and have struggled a lot with stage fright. It was so bad in the beginning that my hands shook off my guitar and I could barely sing. Over the years it's gotten easier, but there are still times when I'm terrified to go on stage. It's taken a lot of strength and bravery for me to go on when I'm feeling so scared. Sometimes the nervousness shifts to a feeling of effortlessness; like I'm deeply connected to the audience and to my bandmates and to an other-worldly stream of music. It's wonderful and has kept me coming back to performing again and again, despite my fears of it. It doesn't matter if I'm in front of five people or one-thousand—some of the most empowering moments I've had have been during or just after a performance that's gone well. It's a subtle thing that can come and go in a flash. I feel a lot of joy and gratitude when somehow everything goes right.*

The birth process usually requires women to encounter external circumstances that aren't in their control. Some of these include the timing and intensity of the contractions, the length of the labor, the amount of effort that is required to push a baby out, complications that may arise from the baby's position, or dysfunctional labors that necessitate the need for medical interventions. No matter how much you plan and prepare, birth can always throw in an unexpected wild card. Empowerment occurs when you maintain an inner sense of self that is committed to serving the process of birthing your baby, no matter what is asked of you. It is showing up with pure intent and the willingness to do what needs to be done. It is the inner experience of "I can; and I will."

> *Empowerment is showing up with pure intent and the willingness to do what needs to be done. It is the inner experience of "I can; and I will."*

Note that empowerment during birthing may manifest either passively when you allow the birth process to unfold or actively when you need to provide the pushing effort to birth your baby. When does empowerment mean being vulnerable and when does it require

114

effort to bring something to fruition? Empowerment may look like the willingness to be open to other possibilities in order to recognize and value the inherent power of flexibility. It can be tremendously empowering to intentionally choose to do something someone else's way. This could be a useful tool to tuck into your back pocket for labor, in case it might be needed.

Knowing how to access your power when you need it is another tool to have in labor. I have identified four steps towards empowerment.

- ❖ Make a sincere commitment. Committing isn't about succeeding or failing—it's about the willingness to give all that you have, if that is what is needed. Sometimes it takes going for broke to figure out the prize wasn't what you thought it was.

- ❖ Accept the responsibility. Ask: "What motivates me to accept the responsibility of birthing and parenting this child?" A laboring woman is an essential participant in the birthing process—she is needed! Remember that it is possible to maintain that responsibility with or without interventions.

- ❖ Trust yourself that you will participate with your best effort. Let your highest part show up for the job.

- ❖ Make a sincere effort to either allow or do what is needed. Trust that this is the most that will be asked of you.

## Self-Confidence

Trusting one's self requires a degree of self-confidence. It is useful to consider how you experience your self-confidence as a woman. Any experience that results in a sense of accomplishment increases your capability for dealing with other life challenges.

✦

*AFTER MY EXPERIENCE OF BIRTHING NATURALLY AT HOME, I felt like a rock star. A sense of euphoria at what I'm capable of (anything!) was permanently engraved on my being from birthing my 9lb, 3:oz, 21-inch son. It deepened my sense of self-trust to profound levels. While I certainly am not always able to carry that elatedness I have noticed a difference in the level of trust and confidence in myself as a parent. I've been sure of myself and my ability from Day One because I did it—nobody else, no drugs—ME. That confidence has built up other parts of my life as well; not just as a parent, but as a whole person. Deeper sense of trust in myself and my ability to stand behind myself—support myself, my intuition, and my decisions.*

One woman who had suffered for years from anxiety attacks chose to birth her baby naturally. In her struggles with the challenges that arose during pregnancy and labor, she found herself coping in ways that she had never encountered before. When she discussed her anxiety attacks after the baby's birth, she expressed that they didn't have the same hold over her that they had previously. Her self-confidence had grown through the experiences of the last year and continued to aid her in her capacity to cope with the attacks.

In order to shed light on your confidence-building experiences, ask yourself, "What is the most challenging thing I've ever done physically or emotionally? What motivated me to persevere? What helped me to cope?" Often these events were difficult and may have involved painful experiences. It is especially important to examine attitudes about any emotional wounds or scars. Do you see them as weaknesses or as powerful lessons that have helped you to grow into a better human being? You birth with the whole of yourself. The more that you can convert your perceptions of past traumatic events into valuable learning experiences, the stronger you become in your ability to cope the next time you are challenged.

*Being ready isn't always necessary before you jump in and start swimming. You can still be empowered even if your ducks aren't all in a row.*

116

Another aspect of self-confidence is the source that you turn to for validation. If you rely on other people's approval it undermines the security that true self-confidence brings. If you turn to your own internal validation you know when you have done the best you can, bringing you to a sense of satisfaction. This may be important if the birth process or outcome doesn't turn out the way you envisioned it.

When women are left with unresolved issues about their birth experiences, they may deluge pregnant women with birth horror stories or tales of breastfeeding nightmares. The fact that they are so dissatisfied is unfortunate. However, it may be better to process their feelings with their birth attendant or a trained counselor than with pregnant women about to have their own experiences. If you are pregnant and someone corners you with a story that is making you uncomfortable, feel entitled to stop her or him. You can explain that it isn't useful for you to hear about negative birth drama, but you would be interested in what was wonderful about the experience or positive ways that she or he coped with the challenges.

*You don't know what you're really capable of until you're pushed to the edge and beyond into your unknown capabilities.*

Sometimes it is tempting to put off doing something until everything is set. Despite all of your preparations, birthing or parenthood may present you with situations for which you are not ready. For example, if you've never taken care of a newborn baby before it may seem so daunting that you wonder if you have what it takes to be a good parent. Consider the possibility that, maybe, it's meant to be that way. Then you have the opportunity of understanding that being ready isn't always necessary before you jump in and start swimming. You can still be empowered even if your ducks aren't all in a row.

Self-confidence involves trusting your capabilities and power in both familiar and unknown circumstances. I tell clients that birth takes you to the edge of yourself and then asks you to jump. Previous life circumstances may or may not have provided opportunities to experience challenges such as intense pain, prolonged fatigue, or unexpected outcomes. These create beliefs and attitudes that act as psychological/

emotional boundaries in regards to your coping capabilities. You don't know what you're really capable of until you're pushed to these edges and beyond into your unknown capabilities. I describe this moment in labor as "leaping off the cliff." When you take this leap, your sense of self matures. The obstacles at the edge of the cliff vary. They might come from fear, the reluctance to really let go, the doubt that your strength will be there when you need it. Likewise, there are a variety of resources that you may call on to make it through that last barrier into the unknown. What reinforces your inner strength? For some women it might be a strong connection to courage, a deep faith in a higher power, the loving support of a partner, or the trust in a birth attendant's guidance.

✦

FOR ME, CONTRACTIONS ROCKED! *Scantily dressed for the brisk morning temperature, I found myself dancing to "Hard Sun" from the "Into the Wild" soundtrack. The coolness of the fresh air, the proximity to outside, and the music all about the great outdoors felt perfect. As the waves became more distinct; pressure, heat, and movement felt necessary and amazing. Contractions were empowering and actually kind of beautiful… feeling my body prepare kept me grounded and in a really positive headspace. Music made my day. I sang with songs and wandered the house, dancing a little, pausing every time a contraction hit to have someone apply pressure and the water bottle to my lower back. I sang to "All I Need"… A gorgeous anthem about having all that it takes to reach for your dreams, on your own. Later, almost naked and on my hands and knees, I moved to the Dixie Chick's "Ain't Going to Make Nice"… another strong song from women choosing their own path, unwilling to give up. "Where is the Love?" by The Black Eyed Peas made us all smile and got me up and moving around the house more. Other than moving and singing, my memory of the day is one of laughter and easy chatter with my husband, my birth team, my sister, and my oldest and best friend.*

*I was fully dilated by 11 am. In reality, I was still kind of waiting for labor to get started. With a fantastic morning under our belt, that's when "it" hit: when I got challenged, when the reality of birthing this sweet babe—of my deepest fears of self-empowerment and realization—*

*truly hit home. After basically "fun" contractions, labor halted. I was, plain and simple, terrified. How the hell was I going to get this baby out? What if I failed? Did I really truly have it in me? Did I have the trust in my own self, my own abilities, my core, my spirit, to do what really, truly needed to be done at this crucial point? Have I ever had to push far, far, far beyond what I thought was possible? I found loopholes of failure in all my experiences of success... I spent the next few hours shut down, in tears, talking to myself out loud in the bathroom, dancing with everyone to techno music, trying to find the genuine willingness that was necessary, and being totally terrified. It took a damn lot of work with my midwife, a really good vomit, and the realization that no one in the world could help me with this. There was no urge to push... in fact, there was an overwhelming urge to scream, "screw it" and bail. But I did get there. After some time alone, my midwife poked her head back into the bathroom and offered something along the lines of "YOU have to choose to birth this baby. Why don't you take ten minutes to gather yourself and then come out, join us, and have your baby." An invitation to do what only I could do. A supportive opening... Ok. I took a breath, or two or three, and I joined everyone back in the family room at the birth chair. Three hours of pushing followed. In retrospect, definitely the hardest thing I have ever, ever done. Pushing seemed to take ten minutes and at the same time ten days. I used my support to an extreme... wide-eyed and in almost disbelief, I remember asking my best friend, "THIS is what you did? It's really meant to work like this?" "All right, people..."is now a phrase that we laugh about in my household. Apparently, between each push, when I found myself ready to go for it once again, that was my call to action for those around me to take my legs, to prepare to brace me, as I readied myself once again to push. And between each and every push, like a broken record, I checked in with my midwife: "This is normal?" "This is working?" "I'm doing ok?" and I kept doing it... (Apparently no one has ever asked her that constantly, that repetitively over three full hours, for that level of reassurance. But damn, it made all the difference for me as I kept on just going for it.)*

*At 5:14 pm my son was born.... Cone-shaped head, hand up by his face, friggin' perfect! I loved the birth chair, and thinking of all the other amazing women who'd birthed on it. I loved holding his little vernix-covered body against mine. I loved the sacred temple-like feeling of my home that day and the weeks following. I loved his huge dark almond eyes when they first opened and looked toward the voices he'd been hearing all those months. He was 6 pounds 10 ounces... a good size for a month early. He was beautiful, tiny, with a head of dark hair. He was here and he was ours.*

*His birth and all of these days following have been profound and deeply beautiful in a way I could never have expected. We are all so lucky... we women who are given the understanding that birth can be beautiful, empowering, natural. During labor I felt a lot of sadness for all the women who labor and birth without true support and encouragement, without the belief that they CAN do this, without the knowing that their bodies are MEANT to do this; that it can be empowering and positive beyond belief. I am relishing the womb-like space created here at our house last week; and am still hesitant to re-enter the bigger outside world. These days I'm left feeling like absolutely anything is possible.*

# Helplessness

The polar opposite of empowerment can be seen as giving up, seeing oneself as a victim or helplessness. One possible solution to a challenge is to escape by letting someone else deal with it. In order to understand how you might be tempted to do this during labor, you might ask yourself, "How do I get out of things when I don't want to do them?" If you choose the victim role you might go into self-pity, get sick, or collapse. People with a strong sense of independence may procrastinate or simply refuse to participate. Those who tend to relate to the world through their emotions may blame someone else for the situation, proceed into panic or hysteria, or attempt to control the situation by playing the drama queen role.

I was attending a woman in labor with whom I had a trusting relationship. I had facilitated her birth preparation class and been with her during her first birth. She expressed herself in a rather vibrant manner. Her first labor had been quick and she had needed a steady presence to ground her when she felt she was "losing it." During the second labor, the level of drama kept escalating as she approached second stage. By the time she had been fully dilated for an hour, she was thrashing about with wrenching moans and had everyone's full attention. Finally, I leaned over, caught her eye and simply said, "More work, less drama." Perhaps because she trusted me, she immediately paused and said, "Oh." She became totally calm and centered and preceded to push her baby out in ten minutes.

The essence of giving up is that it is a way to escape responsibility. Losing touch with your power can be recognized by phrases such as: "I can't do it." "I'm just too tired or weak." "You have to do something about this." The doorway through giving up is empowerment that is manifested by accepting responsibility and participating.

✦

> WHENEVER I THOUGHT ABOUT *an "easier" route, an epidural or c-section, the contractions hurt more. As soon as I brought my focus back to my body and my baby, I was able to get through each contraction one breath at a time.*

The need for unexpected interventions does not mean a woman is escaping her responsibility. Contrast the difference between "I need help," where a woman is still willing to contribute her individual effort, and "rescue me," where she is depending on outside resources to take over the obstacles she is facing. For example, a woman who has been in labor for 30 hours and is still four centimeters dilated is faced with the probability of hours more of work before her baby is born. Both she and her baby are exhausted from the effort they have put in and she still desires to birth vaginally, if she can. This is an appropriate time to recognize that she is not having a normal progression of labor and medicalized interventions may be indicated. Rather than experiencing the use of Pitocin to increase the effectiveness of the contractions and an epidural for pain relief as giving up into failure, she can perceive this decision as needed help to assist her efforts. She remains empowered by being motivated and willing to participate to the best of her ability to do whatever needs to be done to birth her baby. Knowing that she has contributed with one hundred percent effort brings a degree of satisfaction, even if the birth process or outcome is not what she had envisioned initially.

## Moving Beyond the Impossible Point

It is common for laboring women to reach a point where they believe that it's impossible to continue. This is normal. When women feel lost and desperate, they often turn to pain medication because they don't see another way out. While external support from a loving partner, a warm bath, or backpressure is helpful, it often doesn't carry them through the wall they've hit. If they reach out for guidance, what they may get offered is relief from the pain and fatigue with an epidural or narcotics. If they originally had the aim of birthing naturally and end up choosing an epidural before they have fully explored their own inner resources, there is a possibility of decreasing their sense of satisfaction with their own participation in their baby's birth. The use of pain medications largely shifts the locus of control in the birth process to the interventions. There is a difference between choosing an epidural because medical circumstances are necessitating an intervention and choosing it in a normal labor because a woman doesn't see another alternative.

*It is common for laboring women to reach a point where they believe that it's impossible to continue. This is normal.*

✦

THERE WAS A POINT WERE I THOUGHT *it would be impossible. I managed the pain very craftily for phase one—concentrating on pain as a sensation, a function of the brain responding. It was all very well and nice until the transition. Transition was, for me, one searing contraction that effectively obliterated my ability to focus on my pain relieving techniques. I was in a water tub with my husband squatting at my side. I remember feeling very alone and like the pain was too damn much. This was pain of an out-of-control variety. A type that didn't care about my prenatal yoga or acupressure or mental training. I very deeply felt this is impossible. And then, all it once, it transformed. It became a different pain, yelling P-U-S-H.*

*When I waltzed into transition with my second baby, I was better prepared to meet my impossible pain. Although on the outside I was cursing like a sailor, internally I was huddled around my one thought and protecting it from the elements: This pain will end with a baby.*

The piece that often gets overlooked at the "impossible point" in labor is the need for an experienced person to guide you back into realignment with your own inner resources, including your motivation for participating fully in the birth process. This is where your preparation prenatally to formulate your own motivation for empowered birthing pays off. If you find yourself overwhelmed by the challenges of labor, it is often the birth attendant's role to hold your original aim and gently lead you back to it. If you can value what is happening in the labor process instead of avoiding it, your energy moves you forward instead of dragging you back. This is a powerful moment of potential growth when you can become empowered to push through imagined limitations and discover inner resources and strengths that you didn't know you had. If you choose an epidural before you have completely utilized these resources, you close the door on this opportunity—not because you have failed by using the medical intervention but because some

*Stay committed to doing the best you can in every moment and watch the journey unfold.*

part of you may wonder if you might have done more on your own. If, from a deep place inside you, your truth is that you have reached the limit of your inner coping capabilities, then your empowerment is to embrace the pain medications as the right way to do what needs to be done to birth your baby. Stay committed to doing the best you can in every moment and watch the journey unfold.

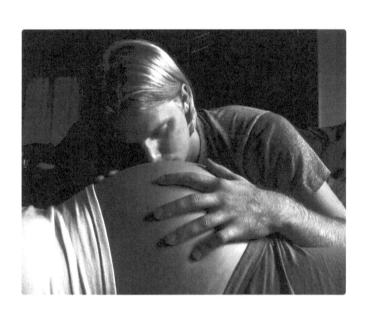

# Receiving and Giving Support

*Sometimes we move on our own energy.*
*Sometimes we get lost and need to be carried for awhile.*

Through the ages, most women have received support from others during labor. Traditionally, this came from other women—mostly mothers, sisters, friends, midwives, doctors, and nurses. This is still true in many cultures. However, around the 1960s more women began turning to their partners as their main labor support person. Before this, most men were not included in the labor and birth process, unless they were in the role of the delivering doctor. For most couples, this change brings a greater sense of wanting to share the experience of bringing their child into the world. Fathers are no longer kept waiting outside until the blood is cleaned up and the baby is happily swaddled in the mother's arms before meeting his new child. Not only is he usually present through the labor and birth; society has given him the role of being the main support person. We're now producing whole generations of men who have far more understanding of the work that women do to birth our babies. Most partners that I work with are quite willing to take on this support role and, at the same time, are often unclear about just what is being asked of them. The most common response when asked why they are attending birth preparation classes is that they want to understand how to support their partner in labor.

FEELING POWERFULLY SUPPORTED *in the birthing environment was crucial to my ability to keep moving forward in the labor process. I really believe that if it had only been my partner and myself, I would have had doubts and been constantly questioning. The sensations were so intense, the pain was so real. But, we did prepare. We had a doula coaching us. We had an incredible nurse. Between these two women (and occasionally, my midwife) their support felt serious and loving; and it felt like truth. All I could do was trust and move forward. The positive culture in the room (that everything was going great even if it didn't FEEL great) made it possible to just put one foot in front of the other (even when the doula made me walk the stairs to move things along!)*

An important point to acknowledge here is that not all partners are men. Particularly with the development of assisted conception, many lesbian and gay couples are choosing to become parents. While the male pronoun is used throughout this chapter, it is done to facilitate the flow of words and not with intent to ostracize female partners. Exploring what support in labor might mean is applicable to any partner, regardless of gender.

Another point is that not all pregnant women have partners. This may be an intentional plan, a result of a relationship breakup or a situation where a woman's partner may not be available when she goes into labor. Most women who face this situation choose to have someone else with whom they are in a close relationship serve as their main support person. Having someone in the room who loves her in a personal

*Having someone in the room who loves her in a personal way is important to most laboring women.*

way is important to most laboring women. It doesn't necessarily need to be a life partner and lover. While friends or family members may love her in a different way than a partner, their relationship can still provide that deep nourishment that helps to fuel a woman through the long hours of labor. While I use the term partner throughout this chapter, other people who are filling the main support role can also utilize most of what is said.

One of the first places to start in working together for birth preparation is for you to formulate just why it is important to have your partner with you during labor. Then, at a time when you both can give it your full attention, communicate that important piece of information to him. Couples often assume that they will both be present at the birth of their children, but there is much more to say than that. Telling him why his presence is valuable to you helps him begin to understand how his role as the support person might unfold. It also helps to honor the special place in the birthing room that is his. Explaining that you want him to push on your back during a contraction doesn't feel the same as saying that you want his arms around you if you get frustrated and lost.

✦

I COULD NOT HAVE HAD AS WONDERFUL AN EXPERIENCE *as I did without my husband. He timed my contractions, kept my mother at bay, and gave me the verbal and physical encouragement I needed, when I needed it.*

The societal shift that has resulted in giving the partner the role of main support person in labor can have a significant affect on your relationship as a couple. Laboring together has the potential to strengthen your bond by deepening one another's respect and appreciation for each other. It also can bring to light difficulties in the relationship, such as a lack of dependability or miscommunications. The more such issues can be addressed before labor, the greater is the chance that your partnership will grow in a positive direction. If you are having relationship difficulties, pregnancy may be an appropriate time to seek the services of a professional councilor. Becoming parents together has the potential to accentuate unresolved issues more than it makes them magically go away. Learning how to best support one another goes a long way in preparing for an optimal birth and parenting experiences.

◆

*WHEN I FOUND OUT I WAS PREGNANT, I knew I wanted to have a homebirth. My husband was a little bit skeptical. He was concerned about safety since homebirth was a new idea to him. I told him to keep all his safety questions and ask the midwives, since I had already made a consultation. When the midwives were able to sufficiently answer all his questions he felt comfortable with us having a homebirth. He was a little nervous about what his role would be during the birth. We attended birth classes, and I let him know that all I really needed was for him to be there. When the time came, he got the birth tub ready and stayed right by my side for the whole birth. The birth went perfectly, and he is now the biggest proponent of homebirths I know. He called everyone he knew and relayed our birth story over and over, telling them how awesome it was to have your baby at home. He loved that our baby was born right in our living room, next to the fireplace and the Christmas tree, and he saw how our baby made such a smooth and easy transition into the world. I love listening from the other room when he's on the phone dramatically describing the birth, and how impressed he was with me and our amazing midwives.*

## The Roles of the Support Person

The sometimes-long hours of labor often require subtle, but important, shifts in the role of the support person. It is difficult to predict exactly what you will need because the challenges of your birthing journey may change in the various experiences you will encounter along the way. You may be striding confidently along at one point and, later, it may take every fiber of your being to take the next step forward. The support you receive from you partner is much more valuable if it has the flexibility to match your needs and moods. The following is a description of some of the roles that your partner may be asked to play, as together you explore what works best in each part of the labor.

*What women usually need most from their partner during labor is to be loved. Women can move mountains when they feel loved.*

# The Beloved

What women usually need most from their partner during labor is to be loved. Women can move mountains when they feel loved. If the two of you are fortunate to have a healthy relationship, your partner usually has some experience in being your beloved. He probably knows you better than anyone else. From your life together, he's seen what often helps you to get unstuck—humor, a reminder of why you wanted to do this, encouragement, leaving you alone to work it out, consolation, a hug, telling you he loves you. Being bathed in a love you can trust is a source of nurturing and strength when you are being asked to manifest the all-encompassing effort that labor may require. The role of the beloved is usually unique to a partner relationship. While other members of the birth team may offer valuable support, it is different than the emotional intimacy that is the core of a committed partnership.

# The Companion

Most women don't want to labor and birth alone. Sometimes pain can feel isolating and bring you to a lonely place. When you are reminded that you are not alone it may help bring you back from a feeling of being lost. It is a big event and having your life partner there by your side usually feels right. Typically, you will both be facing the changes that a child will bring to your futures. Participating together in the effort to bring your baby into the world is the beginning of the expansion of your family. There may be times when you close your eyes and need to turn your focus inwards, when you don't want touch or talking. However, usually when you labor like this, you want your partner sitting next to you throughout the contraction and to be there when you open your eyes. His presence matters, and even when your eyes are closed you may still feel and desire his connection.

I THOUGHT I WOULD WANT *my husband to massage me and be in the pool with me, so I was surprised when I kept on saying, "Don't touch me, don't touch me, just stand here with me," while I hung on to him. His touch felt like adding a hundred extra pounds of pressure to the contraction, and just pushed me over the edge of what I could handle.*

## The Witness

Women often need someone to witness their efforts, to know just how hard they are working, and to express appreciation for it. While your partner can't share the physical sensations that you are feeling, he can walk beside you and share the journey. If you are feeling overwhelmed by what you are being asked to do, you may need to express that and to have someone else who sees the enormity of what you have accomplished. It is important for him to differentiate between your statements about pain, fatigue, and effort being a need to be heard and acknowledged verses a request for him to save you. "This is really hard and it hurts like hell!" may mean that you just need him to know that and doesn't necessarily mean you want him to do something about it. An answer that might satisfy you is, "It looks really hard and you are amazing to be doing it!"

> *Women often need someone to witness their efforts, to know just how hard they are working, and to express appreciation for it.*

## The Consoler

One of the most tender roles that your partner can play during labor is that of the consoler. Because of your lover relationship, he is usually the safest harbor in which to shelter when you face the levels of physical and emotional vulnerability that birthing can bring. He is the person with whom you are most comfortable being physically naked when you find yourself in a room with your birth team gazing at your vagina as you push your baby out. The freedom to vocalize sounds during contractions is a freedom you may have experienced in your sexual relationship together. You may become so frustrated by the challenges you are facing in labor that you begin sobbing from a place deep inside yourself. You may not have ever cried so deeply. For most women, it is their partner's arms they want around them at this moment. It is his chest that you want to turn your face into, to be held until you can get on your own two feet again. Some couples spend their whole lives together and never get a chance to do this.

## The Guide/Rock

Women sometimes lose their way in labor and forget why they are doing this. The pain and fatigue can feel so big that they take over all of your awareness. A simple reminder such as, "That last contraction brought you one step closer to holding our baby in your arms," may be all you need to get your focus back and face the next wave of pain. When your partner plays the role of the stabilizing force it helps you to stay grounded. He can hold the big picture for you both and, at the same time, filter out the distractions that are annoying for you to have to deal with. It can be a little tricky to find the balance between guiding and respecting your self-reliance. Laboring women often don't like being told what to do and may snap back with irritation at suggestions. It is important that he not take your response personally and, instead, try another approach. Rather than telling you to breathe, he can focus on taking deep, audible breaths himself. It always surprises me how often women respond with slow, calm breaths. Guiding with subtlety is an art. The more he can understand how you plan to cope in labor, the greater are his chances of staying in tune with what might be helpful and what might end up being irritating.

# The Protector

Many men can easily relate to the role of the protector. But, be careful with this one. When people around you are manifesting protection energy, there is an increased likelihood that you will question your own safety. Feeling unsafe is not usually conductive to a smooth, normal progression during birthing. This is particularly evident in hospital births when couples are suspicious of medical interventions. Coming in wearing boxing gloves tends to generate an atmosphere of adversity and defensiveness with the birth team that is rarely helpful. In this situation, sugar often works better than vinegar. Diplomacy skills may be subtler but are usually more effective. When your partner provides the social lubrication, you don't have to worry about everyone in the room getting along and can focus on your own work. Simple acts like asking the nurse how her day is going goes a long way in getting her to stretch a few protocols when you're wanting a bit more freedom in labor. I have seen obstetricians suddenly soften when they are thanked for getting up in the middle of the night to perform a cesarean delivery. When they walk into the room of a client who is facing an unwanted cesarean

*An important part of the protector role is differentiating between when he is protecting and when he is rescuing you from something that is your work to do.*

they are often treated as the enemy. Instead, when they are welcomed onto the birth team they feel appreciated. This friendly gesture can change the whole tone in the room and is a step towards creating a positive birth experience, even when it wasn't what you had planned.

Another important part of the protector role is differentiating between when he is protecting and when he is rescuing you from something that is your work to do. This can become particularly challenging if you are struggling to cope with pain, fatigue, or the effort of pushing. If he is unclear about how to respond or interpret what's going on it's useful to pull aside someone on the birth team and ask for guidance. They've seen a wide range of similar behavior and are usually more experienced in how to deal with it.

***Advice from four new fathers
about being in the labor support role***

✦  *Don't tell her she's almost done.*

✦  *Just watch her and follow her cues.*

✦  *Labor takes more endurance than most
men expect.*

✦  *Don't ask her to make decisions—just make
suggestions about what to do next.*

## Potential Issues Around Support in Labor

What if you want to labor alone? Some women retreat into themselves and are clear about their message of, "Leave me alone; I can do it myself." The questions that your support person and the rest of the birth team need to ask are, "Is your isolation working for you?" and "Is labor progressing in a reasonable manner?" If the answers to both these questions are, "Yes," then the best support that they can provide is to minimize distractions and to be there to catch a baby when you're ready to push. What works for you takes priority over maintaining a more obvious connection with everyone else. However, this doesn't mean they should desert or ignore you. Having your partner and team aware of your efforts and ready if you want them may be all the interaction you need.

✦

*During labor I wanted absolute quiet and no distraction. Birthing was really, really personal for me even though I had about ten friends and the midwives all gathered around. I did not want to be touched, held, or even checked by the midwives for that matter. If anyone spoke, I just wanted brief words of encouragement and nothing more.*

If, on the other hand, your isolation is not working for you and you are struggling to cope or labor is not progressing normally, then something else is required. If you are someone who prefers to work alone, it may take some honesty on your part to recognize if things aren't working. For those around you it can feel like you have barricaded yourself behind an emotional door and we can't reach you until you open it. It is wisdom, not failure, to receive help when you get stuck. The support of your partner or advice from your birth team may carry you across a threshold to a path that you couldn't reach on your own. For some women this is easy, and for others reaching out may be the hardest thing they do in labor.

Most people that I work with say that they are more comfortable giving support than receiving it. You keep more control in a situation when you are the giver rather than the receiver. If you are someone who perceives yourself as independent and self-sufficient, it may be challenging to view accepting needed support from your partner or guidance from a birth attendant as a strength and not a weakness. It is possible to find the balance between self-reliance and the vulnerability of openness and connection.

✦

> I FOUND OUT HOW MUCH I NEEDED SOMEONE. *I had to deal with a lot to finally ask my husband to help. It was really the first time I did that. To really take comfort in someone wanting to help me and to have someone there whom I really could trust to help me. My husband was amazing, and we feel there is nothing we can't do together. Our relationship has been taken to a deeper level than we ever thought possible.*

No relationship is foolproof. What if your support person isn't perfect? He may make an honest mistake and misread what kind of support you need or miss your cues that you need support at all. Or it may be that he is tired and overwhelmed and falls into an annoying habit that you have never particularly appreciated. When women are in the thick of labor they are commonly rather short on patience when their partner doesn't get it right. Expending effort to be polite in how you respond to this may just seem like too many balls in the air with everything else that's being asked of you. It may be that all you can get out during a contraction is, "Don't friggin touch me there!" This is a set up for hurt feelings on one side and guilt on the other. One way to possibly avoid this scenario is to agree between the two of you before the birth that labor land is an "offense-free zone." That means that nobody is keeping score of who wronged whom. If you get snappy and irritable, your support person can try something like, "I don't seem to be getting it quite right. Is there something that would work better for you?" This needs to be said in as clean a way as possible without hidden agendas.

*Letting go of doing labor perfectly as a couple is much more like real life than the romanticized fantasy of everyone doing exactly the right thing at exactly the right time.*

Letting go of doing labor perfectly as a couple is much more like real life than the romanticized fantasy of everyone doing exactly the right thing at exactly the right time.

A fairly common mistake that partners can make is to supply the support that they would want, while missing the fact that it isn't working for the laboring woman. We don't all want the same thing when we're feeling stressed or overwhelmed. We also don't necessarily communicate what we need in the same way as others. Before labor begins, it is helpful to sit down together and explore how each of you seek and give support. What works for you and how do you communicate your needs? While you can never completely predict what might come up for you in labor and what your partner's best response could be, it is useful to at least give him a place to start. Be as specific as possible about what you might want, including: the kind of touch, degree of privacy or self-reliance, use of words for reassurance or guidance, making jokes, silence verses chit-chat. Do you want him to whisper that he loves you in your ear or give you a kiss on the back of your neck? How will he know when he's got it right, when he needs to try something else, or when he needs to back off and give you some space? Ask him the same questions in return. If you are sharing a life together, in all likelihood, at some point he will also need your support and you will be better equipped to provide it.

What has been said so far about support is based on the assumption that you can depend on your partner to be there for you and that he will make the best effort that he can. Unfortunately, this is not always the case for some women facing labor. It may be that the support role is too overwhelming for him; the relationship is so new that you haven't had time to develop a deep trust and connection, or the relationship simply isn't supportive and loving. It is tempting to fantasize that the experience of laboring together might improve things between you both. While this is a possibility, labor is not the time to count on healing a relationship or bringing you closer together. That work needs to be done before labor, if you are both willing. The bottom line is that nothing can get in the way of getting your baby born. This has to be your main focus. It is unlikely that you will have the energy to be distracted by issues around relationship maintenance and deal well with contractions and fatigue at the same time. If your relationship is unstable, it might be wise to have someone else there in the role of the main support person. As long as he isn't creating a negative disturbance, it may work to have him present; but it isn't a great idea to count on him. If something wonderful happens and he steps up to the plate with the right connection, it could be an added gift to your birth experience. But be clear with yourself that your service to your baby takes priority.

## Potential Issues for Partners in Labor

One of the most common challenges that partners talk about is seeing their loved-one in pain and distress while feeling helpless to assist her. It may be useful to recognize the difference between supporting you and rescuing you. Birthing your baby is a responsibility that rests on your shoulders and the experience is inside your own body, heart, and mind. There's a limit to how much you share that experience with those around you and how much is for you alone to live. An example of when a partner can get confused about the boundaries between your job and his can arise if you are struggling to cope with contractions or fatigue. You may be starting to talk about considering pain medication and he may jump to the conclusion that he needs to get you an epidural. Choosing an epidural is certainly a valid option, but letting you be the one to discuss that with your birth attendant and make your own choice supports you in staying empowered. He can simply let the birth team know that you are struggling to cope and might be open to a discussion about your options. It's fine to give his opinion if you ask

*When your partner keeps his energy positive about what is happening in labor it helps you to do the same.*

for it. This approach doesn't take over your responsibility and leaves you connected to the process at a particularly sensitive part of labor when there is potential for you to feel that you are losing control.

Many people associate pain, effort, fatigue, and frustration as negative events that are best avoided. In a natural birth, these are all normal events. Partners' attitudes can be influential when women are in the vulnerable world of birthing. When your partner keeps his energy positive about what is happening in labor it helps you to do the same. If he is feeling overwhelmed and unable to contain his doubts or anxieties he may need to take a break to recoup himself. After finding someone else from the birth team to take his place, he can leave for a short nap or food. Sometimes talking with one of the birth attendants about what is concerning him will give him support and help him feel more grounded and safe.

✦

I DIDN'T SEE THE BIRTH *because I was leaning back in the birth chair but I could see everyone around me being joyful and shouting. My favorite moment was looking at my husband who was crying and shouting, as excited as a child on Christmas morning, shouting, "Here she is, here she is!"*

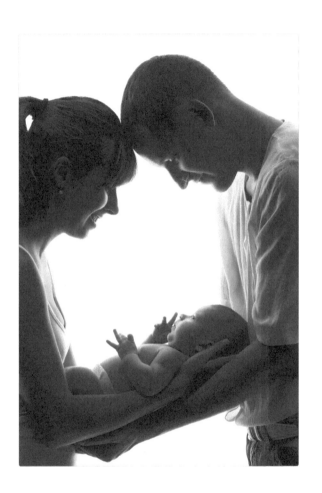

力

# Conclusion

My goal in this book has been to assist women to birth in a way that leaves them satisfied. Whether or not a woman births naturally in the end is much less important to me than her inner journey along the way. The richness of the birthing experience never ceases to draw me in. Birth is real. It matters. For me, it is a micro world where effort, joy, pain, and wonder lead into the mysteries of being alive. I feel the hint that the meaning of life is just around the corner.

I would like to offer you one more tool that might be useful in your birth preparation. I tend to use quite a bit of imagery and allegories in my role as a birth guide and midwife. These speak to emotions and feelings that can inspire you in ways that your logical mind can't always reach. Following is a visualization based on viewing your pregnant body as a birthing vessel. You can have someone read it to you during labor or as practice before labor starts. If you are practicing it more than three weeks before your due date, take a moment to explain to your body that the visualization you are about to do is practice for what will take place in the future when it is the perfect time for your baby to be born. Be clear with your body that today is not when labor will actually start. All parts of you agree to be patient and wait until your baby is strong and mature and can enter the world in a healthy way.

Begin with a deep breath, releasing tension, concerns, and disturbances. Bring your attention to your awareness of your body, present in this moment. Feel your body occupying space, holding your baby in a safe place inside you. As the weeks of your pregnancy have slipped by your body quietly has been preparing itself for the day when it will bring your baby out into the world. Your body understands the honor and the responsibility for the effort that will be asked. It knows that its role as a birthing vessel is a privilege.

Now, visualize your body as a clear vessel. Imagine it any color that you choose. Nestled safe inside that vessel your baby is growing, waiting patiently for the day when you will hold him or her in your arms. Sometime close to your due date your body will set aside most of its other tasks and take on the role of a birthing vessel. It may be several hours that you have been aware of the growing waves of birthing energy that are moving within and finally it is clear that they are getting stronger and more distinct. With this come the beginnings of discomfort. Visualize with each contraction that sacred birth energy is being poured into the top of your birthing vessel, slipping down into a pool that rocks you with its undulations. This sacred liquid comes from a higher place than that in which we live our daily lives. Its precious gift is the ability to bring forth a new life to walk upon this planet. It knows how to do this with a wisdom that far exceeds anything that we will ever achieve.

With each contraction, watch as the liquid flows down into the vessel, swirling and dancing, opening all the right parts, going just where it needs to go. Then you see that it has found an opening in the bottom of the vessel. At first, it slowly drips out of this passage, emptying the vessel with each contraction. As time passes more and more fluid is poured in with each contraction and the waves get stronger, pushing against the walls of the vessel with a kind of power that you've never known before. These waves bring pain to the vessel as it struggles to contain an energy that feels bigger than it is. This energy holds the light of the stars, the heat of the sun, the rush of the wind, the deep dark knowing of the earth. There is so much to contain! As the waves get bigger, the passage opens and, now, the energy flows out in a steady stream—building a pathway of entrance to life.

Still more time passes and now, with each contraction, the fluid almost fills the vessel, rolling through with great intensity and the vessel rocks and sways, moaning with the intensity. You begin to wonder: what will happen when so much energy is poured in that the vessel cannot hold it all? Such sacred energy can't overflow and be lost. The brittle walls of my vessel are close to breaking with the force that is pounding through it.

That's when the magic happens. Maybe it's that the heart and the mind get together because they are so moved by the distress of the vessel. They begin singing an ancient song to a secret place that is hidden in every birthing vessel. And in that place something stirs and feels the vessel's need. And it responds by sending its magic deep into the cells of the vessel walls. And this magic reminds the walls that they aren't brittle or weak. It reminds them that their strength lies in their ability to expand and grow bigger around the waves of sacred energy. In fact, no matter how much birthing energy is poured in from above, your magical birthing vessel releases and gets bigger around it. The liquid now is dancing in joy at the freedom you have given it. For this brief time, you contain the sacred energy of creation. The pain is immense and it doesn't matter anymore. This is a moment of wonder in your life. You are part of an ancient dance. You are connected to everything.

The time for surging and pushing comes and the energy continues to pour through you, accompanying you, guiding you, cheering you on. Time doesn't have meaning again until you look down and realize that your baby has slipped out in the river of birthing energy and is looking up into your eyes. This baby will be your closest memory of that magical time because you understand then that while you were dancing with those waves, so was your baby. You two have shared a sacred journey that will bond you forever.

# References

Elliot AJ, Gable S, Mapes R. (2006) Approach and Avoidance Motivation in the Social Domain. *Personality and Social Psychology Bulletin, 32:3, 378-391.*

Elliot AJ, Thrash TM. (2010) Approach and avoidance temperament as basic dimensions of personality. *Journal of Personality,* 78(3):865-906 Jun.

Tallman, N, Herring, C. (1998) Child Abuse and Its Effect on Birth: New Research. *Midwifery Today, 45, March*

Made in United States
Troutdale, OR
04/23/2024